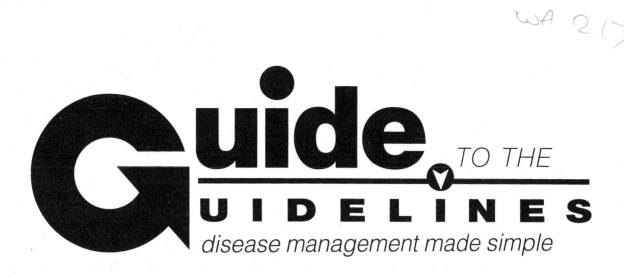

Guide TO THE GUIDELINES
disease management made simple

third edition

Edited by
Peter Smith

Radcliffe Medical

Radcliffe Medical Press Ltd
18 Marcham Road, Abingdon, Oxon, OX14 1AA, UK

First edition 1995
Second edition 1996

Every effort has been made to ensure the accuracy of these
guidelines, and that the best information available has been used.
This does not diminish the requirement to exercise clinical
judgement, and neither the editor nor the original authors can
accept any responsibility for their use in practice.

British Library Cataloguing in Publication Data

A catalogue record for this book is available from the British Library.

ISBN 1 85775 286 4

Library of Congress Cataloging-in-Publication Data is available.

Typeset by TechType, Abingdon, Oxon
Printed and bound by Alden Press, Oxford

Contents

Acknowledgements

This third edition is dedicated to my wife, Linda and my children, Maxwell and Emma. I am eternally grateful to them for tolerating my angst and overwork in preparing this edition during an eventful year.

Thanks again to Radcliffe, for their continuing support and encouragement.

Many of the world's most learned clinicians have spent countless hours preparing the guidelines on which these algorithms are based. Every effort has been made to ensure that the necessary permissions have been obtained to use original material and originating authors and publishers credited. Any oversight is regretted and unintentional – the editor would be pleased to include acknowledgements in future updates if such omissions are brought to his attention.

Introduction

Since writing the introduction to the second edition of this book only a year ago, the term *disease management* has entered common parlance in the medical world. The working definition that I have adopted is: *The development and implementation of treatment programmes for specific conditions in a systematic fashion to optimise the quality and cost-effectiveness of care using the best evidence available.*

In practice, there are probably as many meanings of the term as there are contexts in which it is used. This reflects the fact that there is a continuum of disease management from the development of best practice guidelines to true managed care – a process which encompasses all aspects of healthcare from prevention and education, to primary and secondary care and back to education.

The sudden acceptance of the concept of disease management stems from the many pressures felt within the medical world. Many of the conditions once treated almost exclusively in the domain of secondary care are now managed within primary care, often by teams of professionals rather than exclusively by doctors. As this trend has continued, a need has arisen for a basic level of agreement on therapeutic approach between professionals in both fields. Hence the development of many 'shared care' guidelines.

A further change has been the realization that resources are likely to remain limited, and must therefore be used as effectively as possible. The tendency has been to concentrate on short-term measures covering a small section of healthcare resources rather than on long-term wider benefit. With the increasing devolution of control of total healthcare resources to localities and Total Purchasing Pilots, this need no longer be the case.

At the same time, guidelines on best practice have been issued by accepted 'expert' bodies such as the British Thoracic Society. These tend to be reinterpreted by ever smaller groups of doctors. Rather than contributing to the understanding of the condition, the eagerness of individual doctors to put their own stamp of originality on guidelines has often served to increase confusion.

I have returned to the original sources to prepare these guidelines. Even so, the nature of the guidelines differ. Many are based on the opinions of leading professionals, usually referred to as 'expert' guidelines (e.g. Eczema and Heart failure). Others, such as the Sheffield Coronary Heart Disease Primary Prevention table are purely 'evidence based' and feel almost iconoclastic in their rejection of the cosy myths of accepted teaching. In truth, there is a continuum between Expert and Evidence. A more recent phenomenon has been the increasing use of Delphi consensus techniques for the development of guidelines in areas where evidence is known to be poor, such as the Ontario Knee and Hip Replacement referral guidelines.

This third edition includes new disease areas and updates of existing guidelines. I have also added new references to all disease areas. I hope that this new edition of *Guide to the Guidelines* will serve to assist healthcare professionals in practice and in training in more effective practice of the art of medicine.

Peter Smith
May 1997

List of illustrations

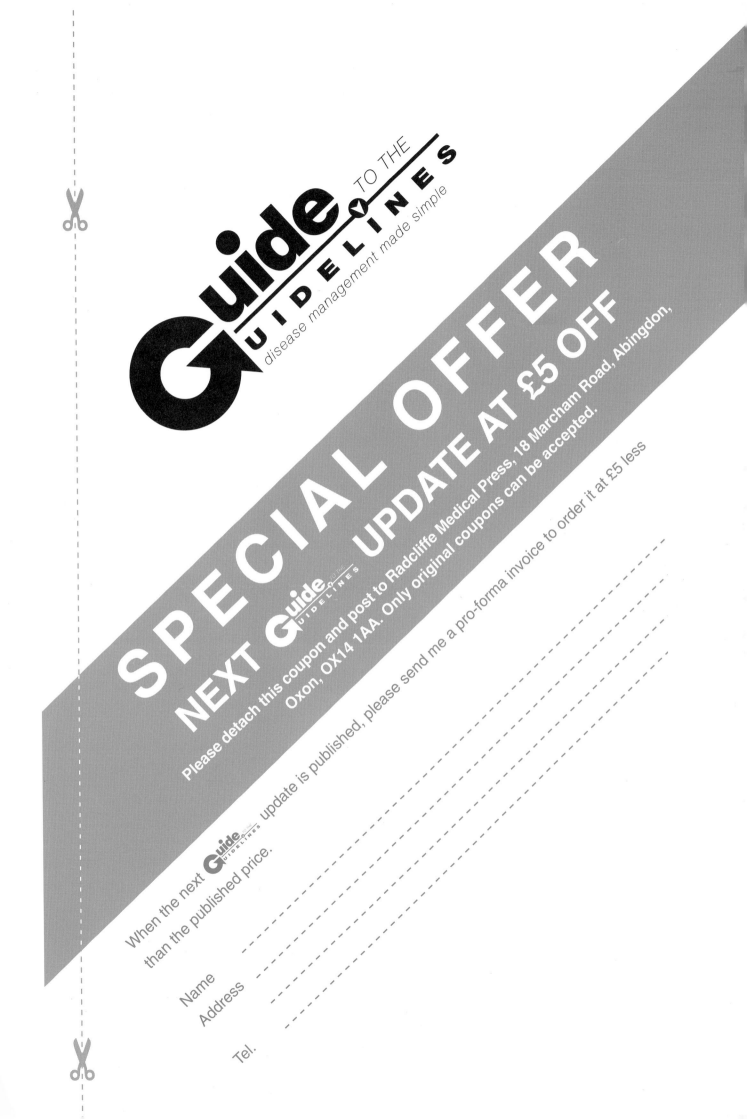

Guide TO THE Guidelines

disease management made simple

SPECIAL OFFER

NEXT Guide UPDATE AT £5 OFF

Please detach this coupon and post to Radcliffe Medical Press, 18 Marcham Road, Abingdon, Oxon, OX14 1AA. Only original coupons can be accepted.

When the next Guide update is published, please send me a pro-forma invoice to order it at £5 less than the published price.

Name

Address

Tel.

Asthma

Chronic asthma in adults and school children

Good practice
Patients should start treatment at the step most appropriate to the initial severity
A rescue course of prednisolone may be needed at any time and at any step
Prescribe a peak flow meter and monitor response to treatment

Essentials for good control
Avoidance of precipitating factors where possible
Patient's involvement and education
Selection of best inhaler device
Treatment stepped up as necessary to achieve good control
Treatment stepped down if control of asthma good

Outcome of steps 1–3: control of asthma
Minimal (ideally nil) chronic symptoms, including nocturnal symptoms
Minimal (infrequent) exacerbations
Minimal need for relieving bronchodilators
No limitations on activities including exercise
Circadian variation in PEFs <20%
PEF 80% of predicted or best
Minimal (or no) adverse effects from medicine

3 **High-dose inhaled steroids or low-dose inhaled steroids plus long-acting inhaled ß agonist bronchodilators**

Inhaled short-acting β agonists as required
Plus either:
beclomethasone or budesonide increased to 800–2000 μg daily, fluticasone 400–1000 μg daily via a large volume spacer or,
beclomethasone or budesonide 100–400 μg b.d. or fluticasone 50–200 μg b.d. plus salmeterol 50 μg b.d.
In a very small number of patients who experience side effects with high-dose inhaled steroids, either the long-acting β agonist option is used or a sustained-release theophylline may be added to step 2 medication
Cromoglycate or nedocromil may also be tried

2 **Regular inhaled anti-inflammatory agents**

Inhaled short-acting β agonists as required
Plus:
beclomethasone 100–400 μg b.d.,
budesonide 100–400 μg b.d. or
fluticasone 50–200 μg b.d.
Alternative: use cromoglycate or nedocromil sodium but if control is not achieved, start inhaled steroids

1 **Occasional use of relief bronchodilators**

Inhaled short-acting β agonists as required for symptom relief are acceptable. If they are needed more than daily move to step 2. Before altering a treatment step, ensure that the patient is having
the treatment and has a good inhaler technique
Address any fears

5 Addition of regular steroid tablets

Inhaled short-acting ß agonists as required with inhaled beclomethasone or budesonide up to 800–2000 µg daily or fluticasone 400–1000 µg daily via a large volume spacer and one or more of the long-lasting bronchodilators
Plus:
regular prednisolone tablets in a single daily dose

4 High-dose inhaled steroids and regular bronchodilators

Inhaled short-acting β agonists as required with inhaled
beclomethasone or
budesonide up to 800–2000 µg daily or
fluticasone 400–1000 µg daily via a large volume spacer
Plus:
A sequential therapeutic trial of one or more of:
Inhaled long-acting ß agonists
Sustained release theophylline
Inhaled ipratropium or oxitropium
Long-acting ß agonist tablets
High-dose inhaled bronchodilators
Cromoglycate or nedocromil

Outcome of steps 4 and 5: best results possible
Least possible symptoms
Least possible need for relieving bronchodilators
Least possible limitation of activity
Least possible variation in PEF
Best PEF
Least adverse effects from medicine

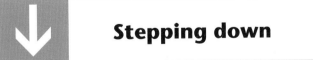

Stepping down

Review treatment every three to six months. If control is achieved a stepwise reduction in treatment may be possible.

In patients whose treatment was started recently at step 4 or step 5 or included steroid tablets for gaining control of asthma; this reduction may take place after a short interval. In other patients with chronic asthma a three to six month period of stability should be shown before slow, stepwise reduction is undertaken.

Asthma in children under 5 years old

Good practice
Patients should start treatment at the step most appropriate to the initial severity
A rescue course of prednisolone may be needed at any time and at any step
(for children under one, 1–2 mg/kg/day; for those aged one to five years,
20 mg/day. Maximum daily dose is 20 mg/day)

3 Increased-dose inhaled steroids

Inhaled short-acting β agonists as required
Plus:
beclomethasone or budesonide increased to 800 μg or
fluticasone 500 μg daily via a large volume spacer. Consider
a short course of prednisolone. Consider adding regular twice
daily long-acting ß agonists or a slow-release xanthine

2 Regular inhaled preventer therapy

Inhaled short-acting β agonists as required
Plus:
cromoglycate as powder (20 mg three to four times
daily), or via metered dose inhaler and large volume
spacer (10 mg three times daily)
or beclomethasone or budesonide up to 400 μg, or
fluticasone up to 200 μg daily
Consider a five-day course of soluble prednisolone (see
notes on good practice above for dosage) or temporarily
double inhaled steroids to gain rapid control

1 Occasional use of relief bronchodilators

Inhaled short-acting β agonists 'as required' for symptom
relief, not more than once daily. Before altering a treatment
step ensure that the patient is having treatment, the inhaler
is appropriate and inhaler technique is good. Address any
concerns or fears. Mildest case may respond to oral ß
agonists

4 High-dose inhaled steroids and bronchodilators

Inhaled steroids (up to 2 mg/day) and other treatments as in step **3**. Slow release xanthines or nebulized β agonists

⬇

Stepping down

Regularly review the need to decrease treatment and step down as indicated. Monitor all changes in treatment by clinical review.

Acute episodes or exacerbations of asthma in young children

Features of mild to moderate asthma

ß agonist therapy: up to ten puffs by MDI plus spacer with or without facemask at one puff every 15 to 30 seconds or by nebulizer every three to four hours

Responds favourably:
- respiratory rate reduced
- reduced use of accessory muscles
- improved 'behaviour' pattern

Repeat every three to four hours
Consider doubling dose of inhaled steroids[1]

Unresponsive or relapse within three to four hours

If still required every three to four hours after 12 hours[2] start a short course of prednisolone for one to three days at 20 mg/day
Infants under a year should receive 1–2 mg/kg/day
One to five year olds should receive 20 mg/day

Increase frequency of ß agonists; give it as frequently as needed, while seeking further help. Start oral prednisolone and refer to treatment outline in full guidelines

[1] It is common practice to advise doubling of inhaled steroids early in the course of an attack, although there is no evidence for efficacy in young children.
[2] Based on the experience of previous episodes, it is reasonable to commence a short course of prednisolone earlier in an attack than indicated here. The efficacy of prednisolone in the first year of life is poor.

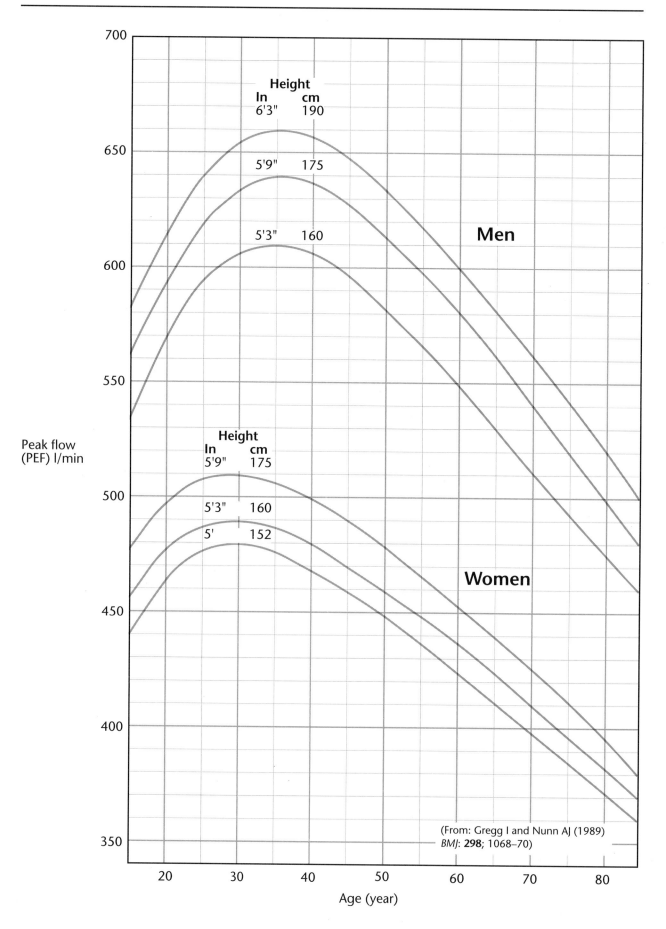

Figure 1.1 Women

Peak flow (PEF) l/min

Figure 1.1 Adult peak flow chart.

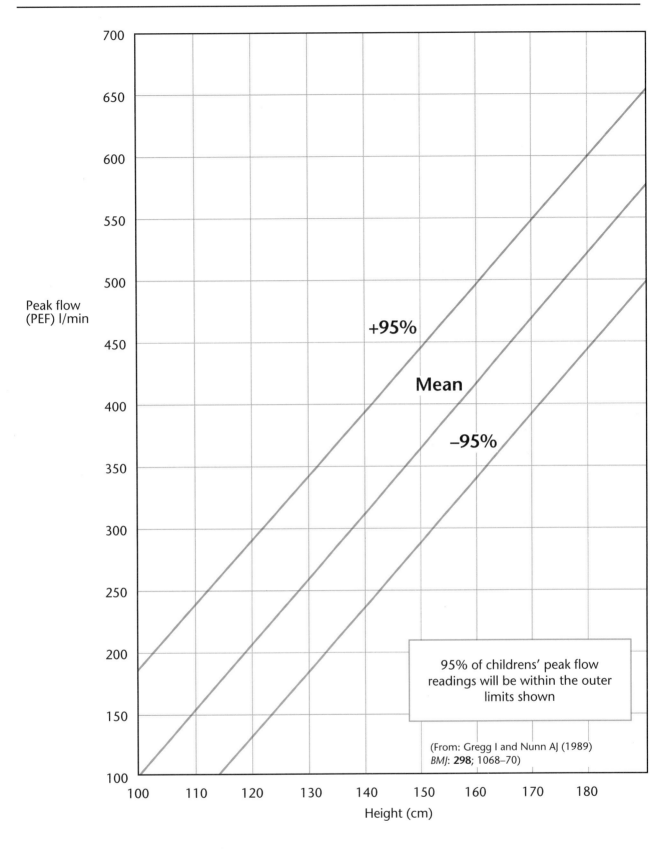

Figure 1.2 Childhood peak flow chart.

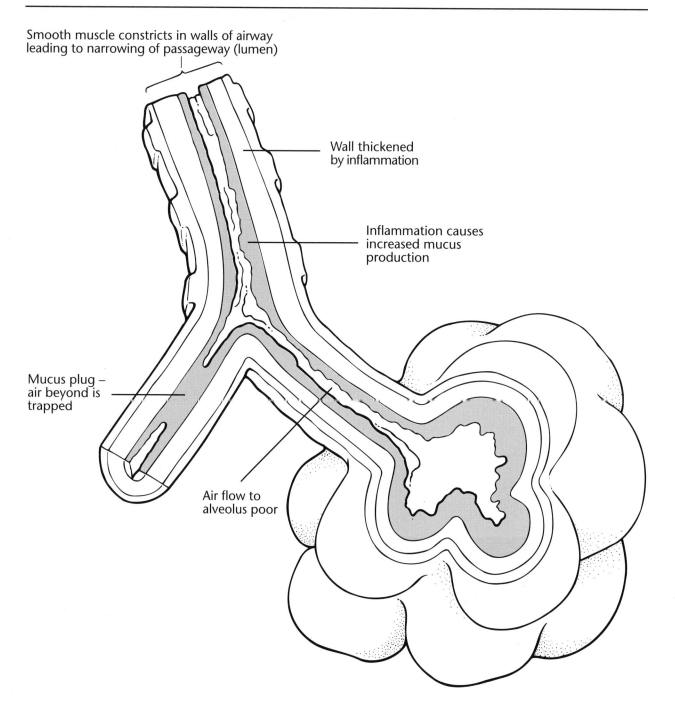

Smooth muscle constricts in walls of airway
leading to narrowing of passageway (lumen)

Wall thickened
by inflammation

Inflammation causes
increased mucus
production

Mucus plug –
air beyond is
trapped

Air flow to
alveolus poor

Figure 1.3 Effects of asthma on airways and alveoli.

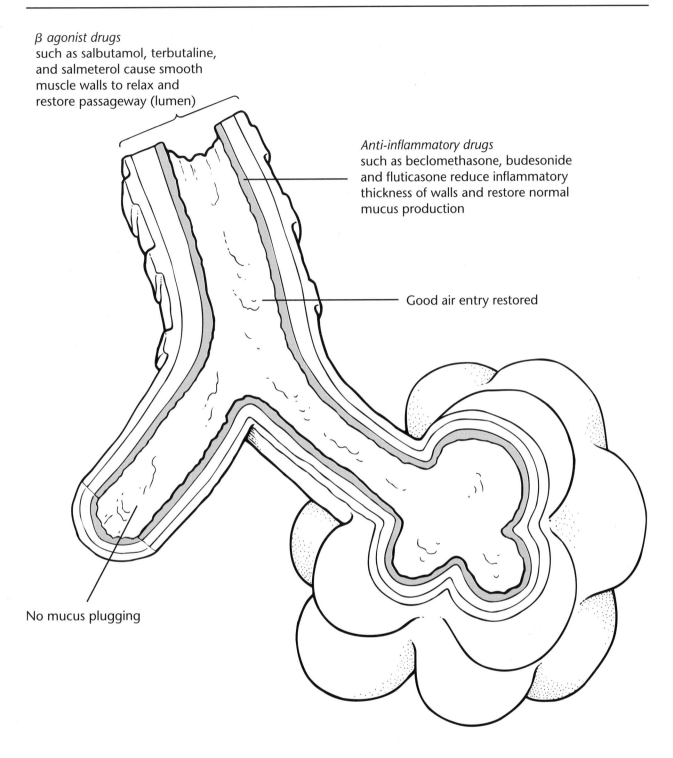

β *agonist drugs*
such as salbutamol, terbutaline,
and salmeterol cause smooth
muscle walls to relax and
restore passageway (lumen)

Anti-inflammatory drugs
such as beclomethasone, budesonide
and fluticasone reduce inflammatory
thickness of walls and restore normal
mucus production

Good air entry restored

No mucus plugging

Figure 1.4   Effects of anti-asthmatic drugs.

Asthma references

This guideline is taken from:
British Asthma Guidelines Coordinating Committee (1997) British guidelines on asthma management : 1995 review and position statement. *Thorax:* **52**; S1-24.

Archer INJ and Simpson H (1985) Night coughs and diary care scores in asthma. *Arch Dis Child:* **60**; 473–4.

Britton MG, Earnshaw JS and Palmer JB (1992) A twelve month comparison of salmeterol with salbutamol in asthmatic patients. European Study Group. *Euro Resp:* **5**; 1062–7.

Centre for Health Services Research (1996) *The primary care management of asthma in adults. North of England evidence based guideline development project.* Centre for Health Services Research, University of Newcastle-upon-Tyne.

Committee on the Safety of Medicines (1992) *Report of the Beta Agonist Working Party.* Medicine Control Agency, London.

Haahtela T, Jarvinen M, Kava T *et al.* (1991) Comparison of a β_2 agonist, terbutaline, with an inhaled corticosteroid, budesonide, in newly detected asthma. *N Engl J Med:* **325**; 388–92.

International Paediatric Asthma Consensus Group (1992) Asthma, a follow-up statement. *Arch Dis Child:* **67**; 240–8.

Lask B (1992) International consensus report on the diagnosis and management of asthma. *Clin Exp Allergy:* **22** (suppl); 1–72.

Rand CS, Wise RA, Nides M *et al.* (1992) Metered-dose inhaler adherence in a clinical trial. *Am Rev Respir Dis:* **146**; 1559–64.

Sears MR, Taylor DR, Print CG *et al.* (1990) Regular inhaled beta-agonist treatment in bronchial asthma. *Lancet:* **336**; 1391–6.

Statement by Thoracic Society Research Unit of the Royal College of Physicians of London, King's Fund Centre, National Asthma Campaign (1990) Guidelines for the management of asthma in adults. 1–Chronic persistent asthma. *BMJ:* **301**; 651–3.

Statement by Thoracic Society, Research Unit of the Royal College of Physicians of London, King's Fund Centre, National Asthma Campaign (1990) Guidelines for the management of asthma in adults. 2–Acute severe asthma. *BMJ:* **301**; 797–800.

Warner JO, Götz M, Landau II *et al.* (1989) Management of asthma: a consensus statement. *Arch Dis Child:* **64**; 1065–79.

Back Pain

Back pain

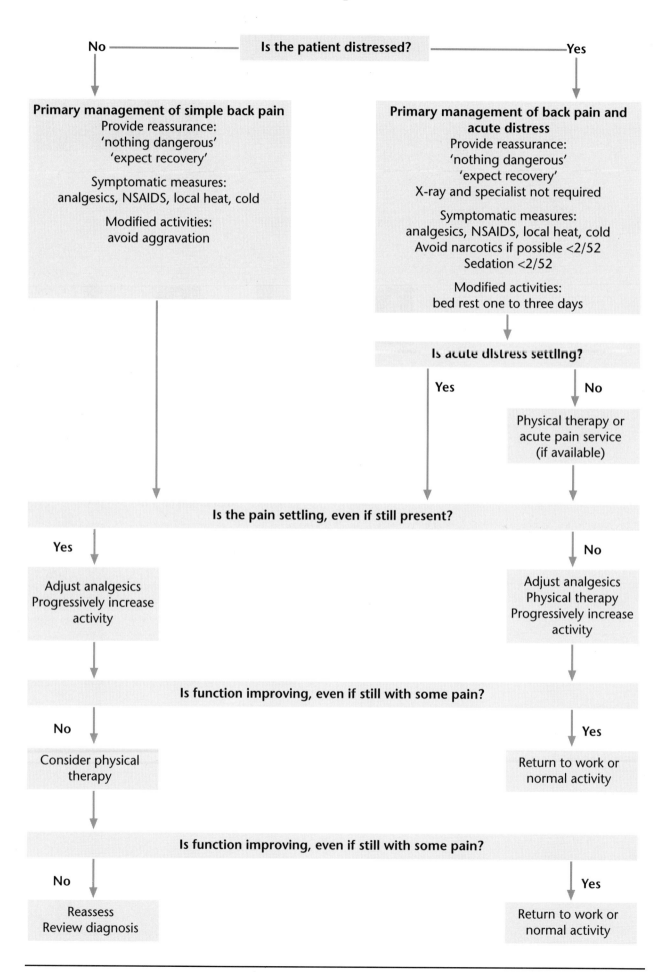

Is the patient distressed?

No ——————————————————— Yes

Primary management of simple back pain
Provide reassurance:
'nothing dangerous'
'expect recovery'

Symptomatic measures:
analgesics, NSAIDS, local heat, cold

Modified activities:
avoid aggravation

Primary management of back pain and acute distress
Provide reassurance:
'nothing dangerous'
'expect recovery'
X-ray and specialist not required

Symptomatic measures:
analgesics, NSAIDS, local heat, cold
Avoid narcotics if possible <2/52
Sedation <2/52

Modified activities:
bed rest one to three days

Is acute distress settling?

Yes   No

Physical therapy or
acute pain service
(if available)

Is the pain settling, even if still present?

Yes   No

Adjust analgesics
Progressively increase
activity

Adjust analgesics
Physical therapy
Progressively increase
activity

Is function improving, even if still with some pain?

No   Yes

Consider physical
therapy

Return to work or
normal activity

Is function improving, even if still with some pain?

No   Yes

Reassess
Review diagnosis

Return to work or
normal activity

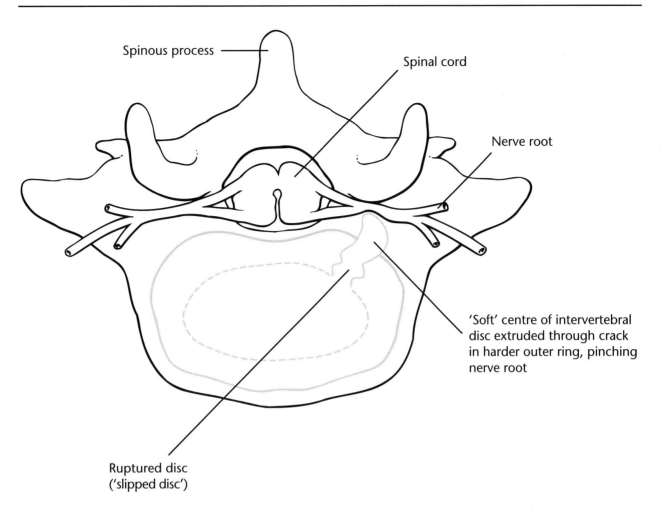

Spinous process

Spinal cord

Nerve root

'Soft' centre of intervertebral disc extruded through crack in harder outer ring, pinching nerve root

Ruptured disc ('slipped disc')

Figure 2.1 Prolapsed intervertebral disc – 'slipped disc'.

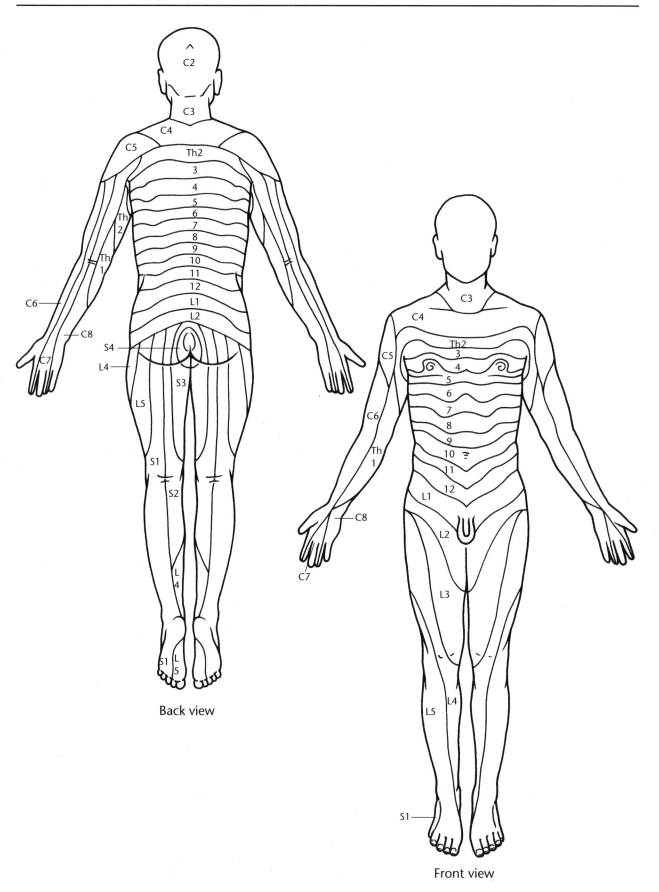

Figure 2.2 Dermatomes.

Back pain references

This guideline is adapted from:
Clinical Standards Advisory Group (1995) *Report of a CSAG Committee on Back Pain*. HMSO, London. Crown copyright is reproduced with permission of the Controller of HMSO.

Davies HT, Crombie IK, Macrae WA *et al.* (1996) Audit in pain clinics: changing the management of low-back and nerve-damage pain. *Anaesthesia*: **51**(7); 641–6.

Deyo RA, Diehl AK and Rosenthal M (1986) How many days of bedrest for acute low back pain? *New Engl J Med*: **315**; 1064–70.

Deyo RA, Walsh NE, Martin DC *et al.* (1990) A controlled trial of transcutaneous electrical nerve stimulation (TENS) and exercise for chronic low back pain. *N Engl J Med*: **322**; 1627–34.

Gilbert JR, Taylor DW, Hildebrand A *et al.* (1985) Clinical trial of common treatments for low back pain in family practice. *BMJ*: **291**; 791–4.

Halpin SFS, Yeonnan L and Dundas DD (1991) Radiographic examination of the lumbar spine in a community: an audit of current practice. *BMJ*: **303**; 813–15.

Hazard RG, Fenwick JW, Kalisch SM *et al.* (1989) Functional restoration with behavioural support. A one year prospective study of patients with chronic low back pain. *Spine*: **14**; 157–61.

Koes BW, Bouter LM, van Mameren H *et al.* (1992) Randomised clinical trial of manipulative therapy and physiotherapy for persistent back and neck complaints: results of one year follow up. *BMJ*: **304**; 601–5.

Linton S, Hellsing AL and Andersson D (1993) Controlled study of the effects of an early intervention on acute musculoskeletal pain problems. *Pain*: **54**; 353–9.

Mayer TG, Gatchel KJ, Mayer H *et al.* (1987) A prospective two year study of functional restoration in industrial low back injury. An objective assessment procedure. *JAMA*: **258**; 1763–7.

Oland G and Tveiten G (1991) A trial of modern rehabilitation for chronic low back pain and disability: vocational outcome and effect of pain modulation. *Spine*: **16**; 457–9.

RCGP (1996) *National Low Back Pain Clinical Guidelines*. The Royal College of General Practitioners, London (also available free on RCGP Internet home page).

Wiesel SW, Feffer HL and Borenstein DG (1988) Evaluation and outcome of low back pain of unknown etiology. *Spine*: **13**; 679–80.

3

Breast Disease

Breast lump

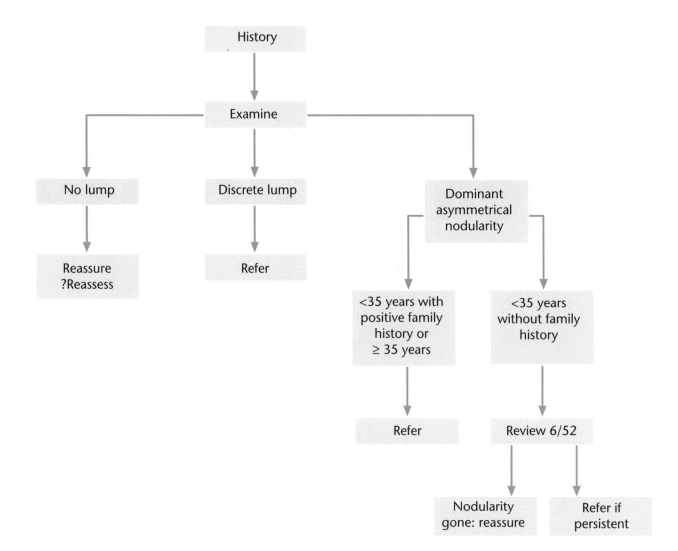

Breast pain

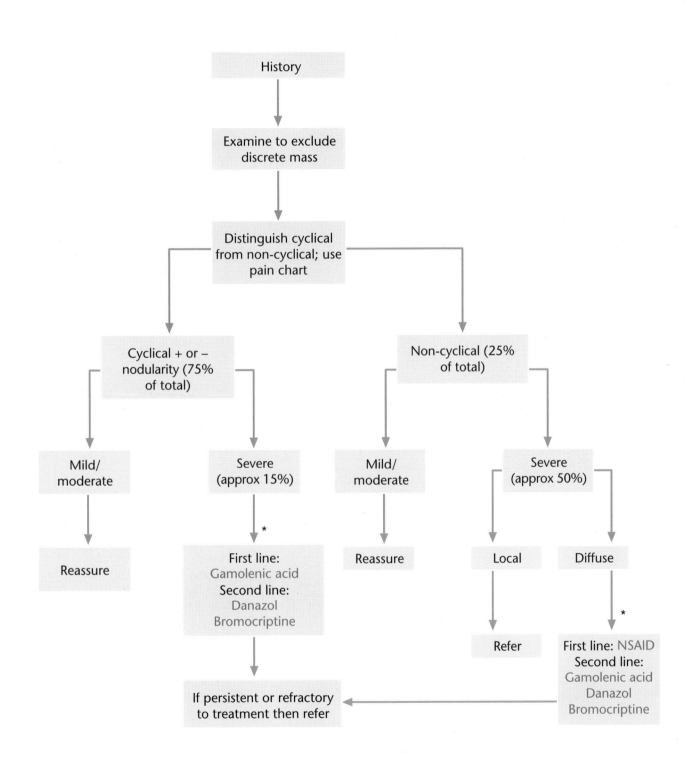

*Local management protocols may differ; please discuss with your local breast unit

Moderate/severe cyclical mastalgia

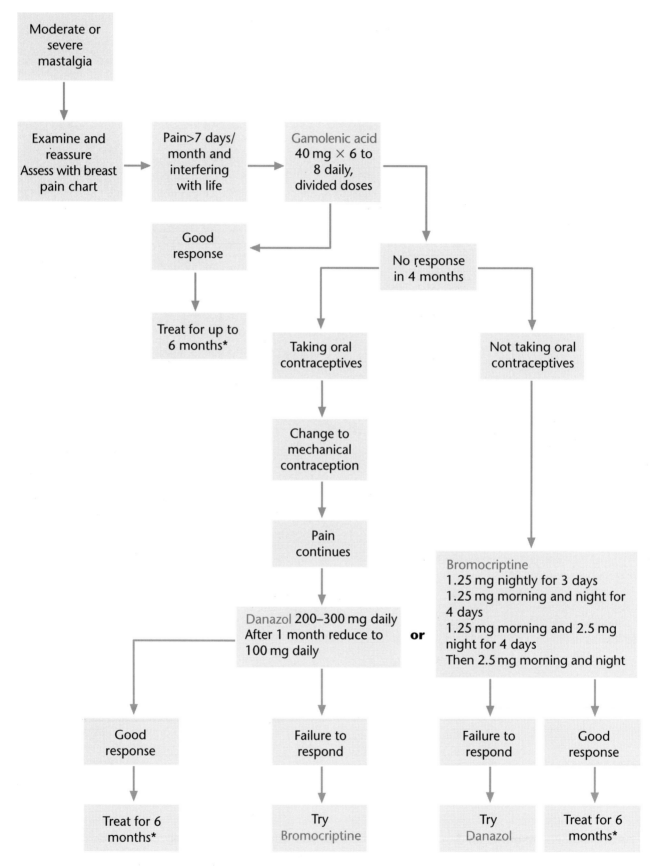

*Stop after 6 months. Half will not require further treatment. If required, repeat previously successful courses of treatment.

Nipple discharge

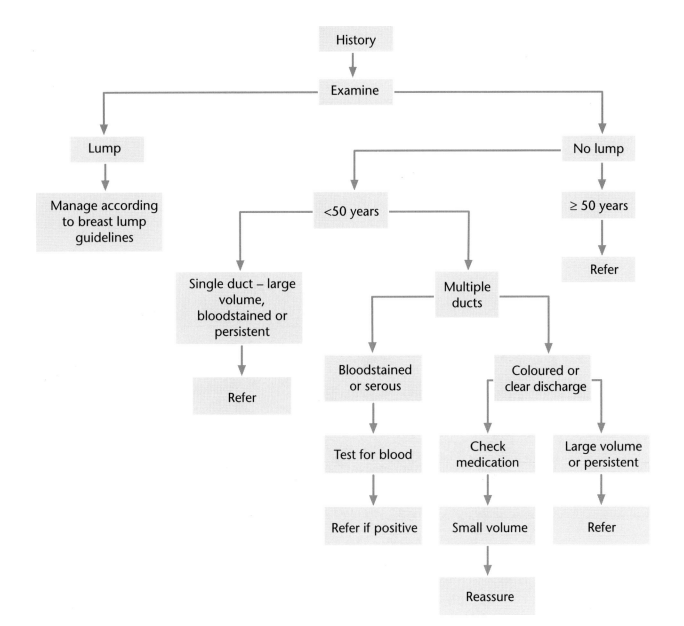

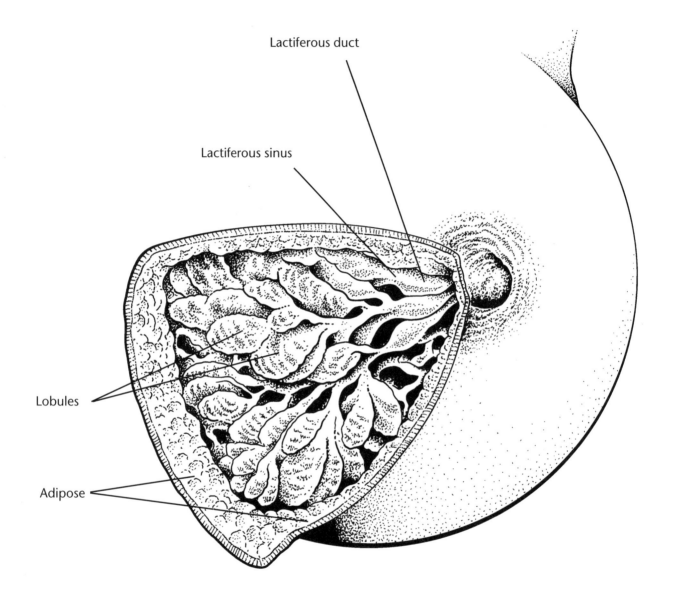

Lactiferous duct

Lactiferous sinus

Lobules

Adipose

Figure 3.1 The breast during lactation.

Breast disease references

This guideline is based on:
Austoker J, Mansel M, Baum M *et al.* (1995) *Guidelines for Referral of Patients with Breast Problems.* NHS Breast Screening Programme, Sheffield.

Bellantone R, Rossi S, Lombardi CP *et al.* (1995) Excisional breast biopsy: when, why and how? *Inter Surg*: **80**(1); 75–8.

Campbell HS, McBean M, Mandin H *et al.* (1994) Teaching medical students how to perform a clinical breast examination. *Academic Medicine*: **69**(12); 993–5.

Curtin JJ and Sampson MA (1992) Need for open access non-screening mammography in a hospital with a specialist breast clinic service. *BMJ*: **304**; 549–51.

Dixon JM, Ravisekar O, Cunningham M *et al.* (1996) Factors affecting outcome of patients with impalpable cancer detected by breast screening. *Brit J Surg*: **83**(7); 997–1001.

Forrest AP, Stewart HJ, Everington D *et al.* (1996) Randomised controlled trial of conservation therapy for breast cancer: 6-year analysis of the Scottish trial. Cancer Trials Breast Group. *Lancet*: **348**; 708–13.

Garstin IW, Kaufman Z, Michell MJ *et al.* (1993) Side-effects of screening. *Euro Cancer*: **29A**(15); 2150–2.

Grunfeld E, Mant D, Yudkin P *et al.* (1996) Routine follow up of breast cancer in primary care: randomised trial. *BMJ*: **313**; 665–9.

Newcomb PA, Storer BE, Longnecker MP *et al.* (1996) Pregnancy termination in relation to risk of breast cancer. *JAMA*: **275**(4); 283–7.

Sandison AJ, Gold DM, Wright P *et al.* (1996) Breast conservation or mastectomy: treatment choice of women aged 70 years and older. *Brit J Surg*: **83**(7); 994–6.

Venn A, Watson L, Lumley J *et al.* (1995) Breast and ovarian cancer incidence after infertility and vitro fertilisation. *Lancet*: **346**; 995–1000.

Cardiovascular Risk Assessment

Cardiovascular risk assessment – primary prevention

The Sheffield Table

This table is based on an extrapolation of the secondary prevention 4S trial into primary prevention, treating those with similar or higher risk. It can be used:

- To identify for primary prevention individuals with a specified coronary risk, in whom treatment with an HMGCoA reductase inhibitor (or 'statin') might be justifiable
- To find the cholesterol concentration for such individuals that confers the specified degree of coronary risk
- To show those individuals who, whatever their cholesterol concentration, will not have a coronary risk that justifies lipid-lowering therapy ('your cholesterol is high, but your risk is low') and therefore do not need screening

Important notes to read before using the table

- Use for decisions on **primary prevention** only. If the patient has a family history of premature CHD and/or hyperlipidaemia, or is known to have a high level of HDL-Cholesterol, measure serum cholesterol level and if raised seek specialist advice
- Left ventricular hypertrophy (LVH) is defined as an increased R-wave potential and flattened or inverted T waves in the left precordial leads
- Use the average of two or more cholesterol concentrations
- Use after appropriate advice on smoking and diet; table assumes that systolic blood pressure in hypertensive patients has been controlled to ≤160 mmHg

How to use the table

- Identify the appropriate column for the presence or absence of hypertension, smoking, diabetes and LVH (LVH can be assumed to be absent if there is no hypertension)
- Identify the row showing the age of the patient
- Read the cholesterol concentration at the intersection
- If there is no number entered at the intersection, cholesterol measurement may be avoided. If the average cholesterol on repeated measurement is at or above the level shown, the absolute CHD event (myocardial infarction or coronary death) risk is ≥ 3.0% per year
- At this risk (3.0% events per year) treatment with a statin should improve outcome

Cholesterol concentration (mmol/L) in men

Hypertension	Yes	Yes	Yes	Yes	Yes	No	Yes	Yes	No	No	Yes	No
Smoking	Yes	Yes	No	No	Yes	Yes	Yes	No	Yes	No	No	No
Diabetes	Yes	No	Yes	No	Yes	Yes	No	Yes	No	Yes	No	No
LVH	Yes	Yes	Yes	Yes	No	No	No	No	No	No	No	No

Age (years)												
70	5.5	5.5	5.5	5.5	5.5	5.5	5.5	5.5	5.5	6.0	6.5	7.7
68	5.5	5.5	5.5	5.5	5.5	5.5	5.5	5.5	5.6	6.4	6.9	8.2
66	5.5	5.5	5.5	5.5	5.5	5.5	5.5	5.7	5.9	6.8	7.3	8.7
64	5.5	5.5	5.5	5.5	5.5	5.5	5.5	6.1	6.3	7.3	7.8	9.3
62	5.5	5.5	5.5	5.5	5.5	5.5	5.6	6.5	6.7	7.8	8.3	
60	5.5	5.5	5.5	5.5	5.5	5.6	6.0	6.9	7.2	8.3	8.9	
58	5.5	5.5	5.5	5.5	5.5	6.1	6.5	7.4	7.7	8.9		
56	5.5	5.5	5.5	5.5	5.5	6.5	7.0	8.0	8.3			
54	5.5	5.5	5.5	5.5	5.9	7.0	7.5	8.6	9.0			
52	5.5	5.5	5.5	5.5	6.3	7.6	8.1	9.3				
50	5.5	5.5	5.5	5.7	6.9	8.2	8.8					
48	5.5	5.5	5.5	6.2	7.5	8.9						
46	5.5	5.5	5.5	6.8	8.2							
44	5.5	5.5	5.8	7.4	9.0							
42	5.5	5.6	6.4	8.2								
40	5.5	6.1	7.1	9.0								
38	5.5	6.8	7.9									
36	6.0	7.6	8.8									
34	6.7	8.6										
32	7.6											
30	8.7											
≤29												

Cholesterol concentration (mmol/L) in women

Hypertension	Yes	Yes	Yes	Yes	Yes	No	Yes	Yes	No	No	Yes	No
Smoking	Yes	No	Yes	Yes	No	Yes	No	Yes	No	Yes	No	No
Diabetes	Yes	Yes	No	Yes	No	Yes	Yes	No	Yes	No	No	No
LVH	Yes	Yes	Yes	No	Yes	No	No	No	No	No	No	No

Age (years)												
70	5.5	5.5	5.5	5.8	6.3	6.9	8.5	9.8				
68	5.5	5.5	5.5	5.8	6.4	7.0	8.6	9.9				
66	5.5	5.5	5.5	5.9	6.5	7.1	8.7	10.0				
64	5.5	5.5	5.5	6.1	6.6	7.2	8.9					
62	5.5	5.5	5.5	6.2	6.8	7.4	9.1					
60	5.5	5.5	5.5	6.4	7.0	7.7	9.4					
58	5.5	5.5	5.5	6.7	7.3	8.0	9.8					
56	5.5	5.5	5.5	7.0	7.7	8.4						
54	5.5	5.5	5.5	7.4	8.1	8.9						
52	5.5	5.5	5.9	7.9	8.7	9.4						
50	5.5	5.5	6.4	8.5	9.3							
48	5.5	6.0	6.9	9.3								
46	5.5	6.7	7.7									
44	5.5	7.5	8.6									
42	5.8	8.5	9.8									
40	6.7	9.9										
38	8.0											
36	9.7											
≤35												

Cardiovascular risk assessment references

This guideline is based on:
Ramsay LE, Haq IU, Jackson PR and Yeo WW (1996) The Sheffield table for primary prevention of coronary heart disease: corrected. *Lancet*: **348**; 1251–2. Reproduced with permission.

Davey-Smith G, Song F and Sheldon TA (1993) Cholesterol lowering and mortality: the importance of considering initial level of risk. *BMJ*: **306**; 1367–73.

EAS Task Force for Prevention of Coronary Heart Disease (1992) Prevention of coronary heart disease: scientific background and new clinical guidelines. *Nutr Metab Cardiovasc Dis*: **2**; 113–56.

Evans P and Pereira Gray D (1994) Value of screening for secondary causes of hyperlipidaemia in general practice. *BMJ*: **309**; 509–10.

Law MR, Wald NJ and Thompson SG (1994) By how much and how quickly does reduction in serum cholesterol concentration lower risk of ischaemic heart disease? *BMJ*: **308**; 367–72.

MAAS Investigators (1994) Effect of simvastatin on coronary atheroma: the Multicentre Anti Atheroma Study (MAAS). *Lancet*: **344**; 633–8.

Oliver M, Poole-Wilson P and Shepherd J *et al.* (1995) Lower patient's cholesterol now. *BMJ*: **301**; 1280–81.

Pyorala K, de Backer G, Graham I *et al.* (1994) Prevention of coronary heart disease in clinical practice: recommendations of the Task Force of the European Society of Cardiology. European Atherosclerosis Society and European Society of Hypertension. *Eur Heart J*: **15**; 1300–31.

Ramsay LE, Yeo WW and Jackson PR (1991) Dietary reduction of serum cholesterol concentration: time to think again. *BMJ*: **303**; 953–7.

Sacks FM, Pfeffer MA, Moye LA *et al.* (1996) The effect of pravastatin on coronary events after myocardial infarction in patients with average cholesterol levels. Cholesterol and Recurrent Events (CARE) Trial. *New Engl J Med*: **335**; 1001–9.

Scandinavian Simvastatin Survival Study Group (1994) Randomised trial of cholesterol lowering in 4444 patients with coronary heart disease: the Scandinavian Simvastatin Survival Study (4S). *Lancet*: **344**; 1383–9.

Shaper AG, Pocock SJ, Phillips AN *et al.* (1986) Identifying men at high risk of heart attacks: strategy for use in general practice. *BMJ*: **293**; 474–9.

Shepherd J, Cobbe S, Fore I *et al.* (1995) Prevention of coronary heart disease with pravastatin in men with hypercholesterolaemia. The West of Scotland Coronary Prevention Study Group (WOSCOPS). *N Engl J Med*: **333**; 1301–7.

Tunstall-Pedeo H (1991) The Dundee coronary risk-disk for management of change in risk factors. *BMJ*: **303**; 744–7.

5

Cervical Cytology

Management of cervical smears

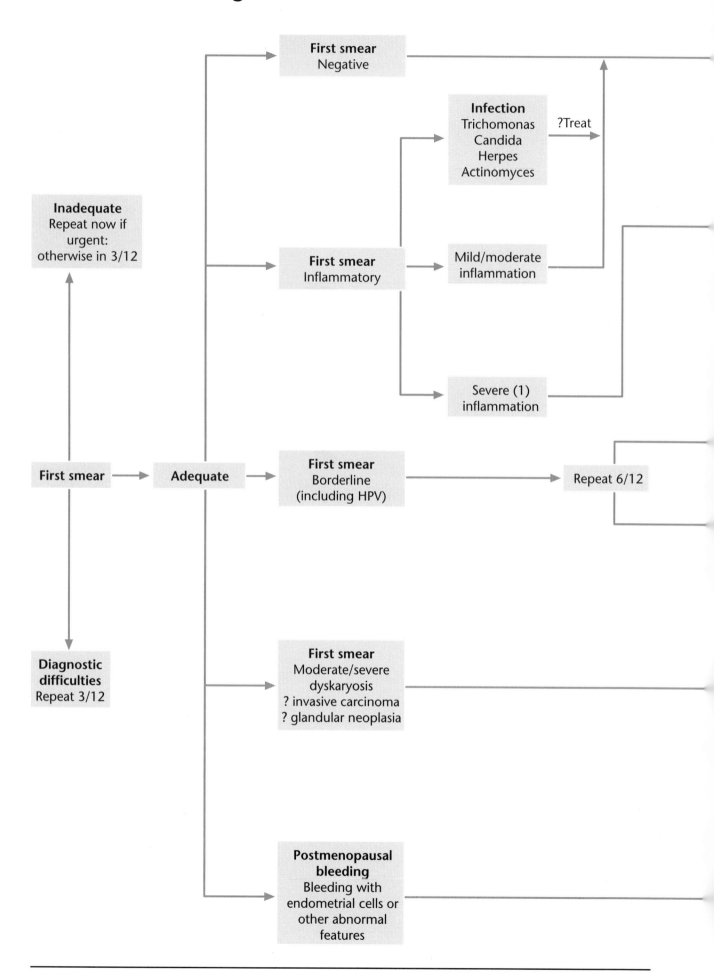

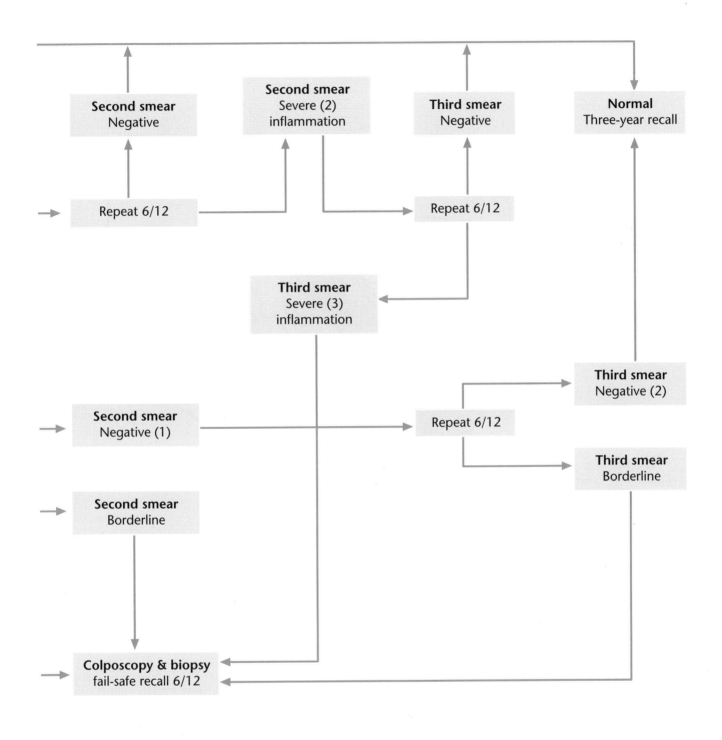

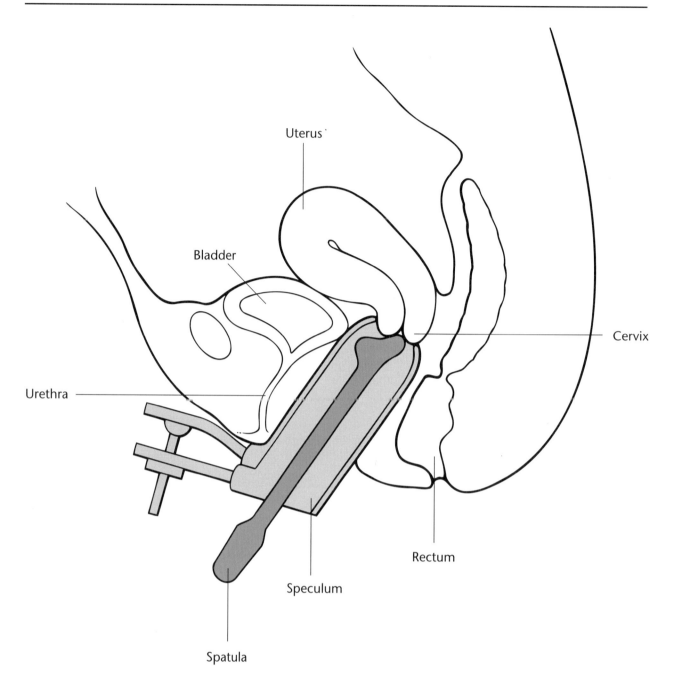

Figure 5.1   Normal female reproductive system showing cervical smear being taken.

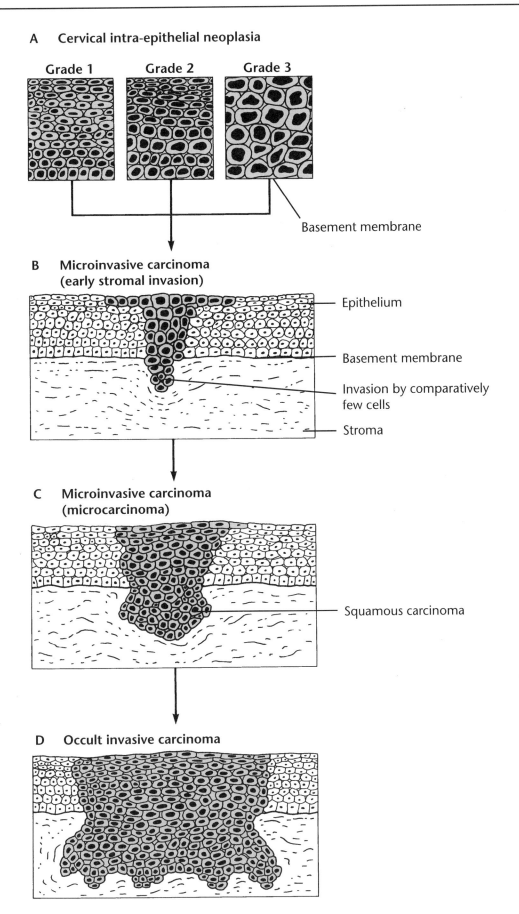

Figure 5.2 Development of carcinoma from CIN.

Cervical cytology references

This is a local guideline developed and used by Charing Cross Hospital and is reproduced with permission from Lant A and Hargreaves S (1993) *Management Guidelines*. Riverside Health (in conjunction with Kensington, Chelsea and Westminster Health Authority).

Anonymous (1993) Cervical cytology: evaluation and management of abnormalities. *I J Gynaecol & Obstet*: **43**(2); 212–9.

Busseniers AE and Sidawy MK (1991) Inflammatory atypia on cervical smears. A diagnostic dilemma for the gynecologist. *J Repro Med*: **36**(2); 85–8.

de Vet HC and Sturmans F (1994) Risk factors for cervical dysplasia: implications for prevention, *Public Health*: **108**(4); 241–9.

Dey P, Collins S, Desai M *et al.* (1996) Adequacy of cervical cytology sampling with Cervex brush and the Aylesbury spatula: a population based randomised controlled trial. *BMJ*: **313**, 721–3.

Flannelly G, Anderson D, Kitchener HC *et al.* (1994) Management of women with mild and moderate cervical dyskaryosis. *BMJ*: **308**; 1399–403.

Jones MH, Jenkins D and Singer A (1992) Conservative treatment of mild/moderate cervical dyskaryosis. *Lancet*: **339**; 1293.

Mayeaux EJ Jr, Harper MB, Abreo F *et al.* (1995) A comparison of the reliability of repeat cervical smears and colposcopy in patients with abnormal cervical cytology. *J Family Practice*: **40**(1); 57–62.

Montz FJ, Monk BJ, Fowler JM *et al.* (1992) Natural history of the minimally abnormal Papanicolaou smear. *Obstet & Gynecol*: **80**(3 Pt 1); 385–8.

Narod SA, Thompson DW, Jain M *et al.* (1991) Dysplasia and the natural history of cervical cancer: early results of the Toronto Cohort Study. *Europ J Cancer*: **27**(11); 1411–6.

Raffle AE, Alden B and Mackenzie EF (1995) Detection rates for abnormal cervical smears: what are we screening for? *Lancet*: **345**; 1469–73.

Regi A, Krishnaswami H, Jairaj P *et al.* (1994) Management of patients with mildly dysplastic cervical smears. *J Repro Med*: **39**(6); 455–8.

Skegg DC (1995) Cervical screening blues. *Lancet*: **345**; 1451–2.

6

Depression

Depression

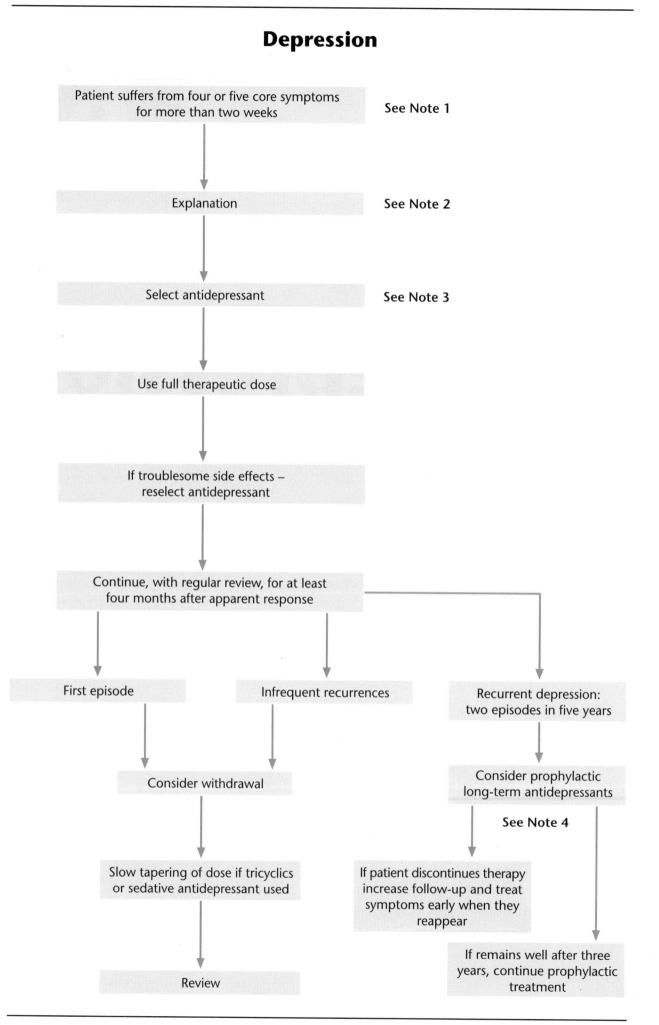

Patient suffers from four or five core symptoms for more than two weeks — See Note 1

Explanation — See Note 2

Select antidepressant — See Note 3

Use full therapeutic dose

If troublesome side effects – reselect antidepressant

Continue, with regular review, for at least four months after apparent response

First episode

Infrequent recurrences

Recurrent depression: two episodes in five years

Consider withdrawal

Consider prophylactic long-term antidepressants

See Note 4

Slow tapering of dose if tricyclics or sedative antidepressant used

If patient discontinues therapy increase follow-up and treat symptoms early when they reappear

Review

If remains well after three years, continue prophylactic treatment

Depression

Note 1 – Core symptoms

Diagnosis can be made if four or five of the following core symptoms have been present for two weeks or more, of which symptoms one and two must be present:

1 Depressed mood
2 Loss of interest or pleasure
3 Loss of energy or fatigue
4 Concentration difficulties
5 Appetite disturbances
6 Agitation or retardation
7 Worthlessness or self-blame
8 Suicidal thoughts

The presence of precipitating factors does not preclude diagnosis or treatment

Depressive symptoms can be masked in the following:

The physically ill
Somatic presentation
The elderly

Note 2 – Explanation

Should include:

'Depression is an illness with an organic basis'
'Effective pharmacological treatment exists'

Reassurance

Psychological and social support

Note 3 – Choosing an antidepressant

If there are suicidal thoughts, the patient lives alone or is at risk, consider using the newer antidepressants

Note that older tricyclics are cardiotoxic, dangerous in overdose and can impair memory and psychomotor function

Note 4 – Long-term antidepressants

To date, the antidepressants that have been shown to be effective long-term include: imipramine, fluoxetine, paroxetine, sertraline, and possibly amitriptyline and maprotiline

Depression references

The algorithm is adapted from the guidelines contained within:
Montgomery SA (1993) Guidelines for treating depressive illness with antidepressants. A statement from the British Association of Psychopharmacology. *J Psychopharm*: **7**(1); 19–23.

Angst J and Dobler-Mikola A (1984) The Zurich study: III diagnosis of depression. *Eur Arch Psychiatr Neurol Sci*: **234**; 30–7.

Beaumont G (1989) The toxicity of antidepressants. *Br J Psychiat*: **154**; 454–8.

Cassidy S and Henry J (1987) Fatal toxicity of antidepressant drugs in overdose. *BMJ*: **295**; 1021–4.

Doogan DP and Caillard V (1992) Sertraline in the prevention of depression. *Br J Psych*: **160**; 217–22.

Freeling P, Rao BM, Paykel ES *et al.* (1985) Unrecognised depression in general practice. *BMJ*: **290**; 1880–3.

Grove WM, Andreason NC, Young M *et al.* (1987) Isolation and characterization of a nuclear depressive syndrome. *Psychol Med*: **17**; 471–84.

Hurry J, Bebbington PE and Tennant C (1987) Psychiatric symptoms and social disablement as determinants of illness behaviour. *Aust NZ J Psychiatr*: **21**; 68–74.

Linde K, Ramirez G, Mulrow C *et al.* (1997) St John's wort for depression – an overview and meta-analysis of randomised clinical trials. *BMJ*: **313**; 253–7.

Montgomery SA (1989) Prophylaxis in recurrent unipolar depression: a new indication for treatment studies. *J Psychopharma*: **3**; 47–53.

Paykel ES (1978) Contribution of life events to causation of psychiatric illness. *Psychol Med*: **8**; 245–53.

Paykel ES, Hollyman JA, Freeling P *et al.* (1988) Prediction of therapeutic benefit amitriptyline in mild depression: a general practice placebo-controlled trial. *J Affect Disord*: **14**; 83–95.

Tylee AT and Freeling P (1988) The recognition, diagnosis and acknowledgement of depressive disorder by general practitioners. In *Depression: an integrative approach* (K Herbst and ES Paykel eds) Heinemann, Oxford, pp. 216–31.

Diabetes –
Non-Insulin Dependent Diabetes Mellitus

Diabetes: diagnosis

Diagnosis of diabetes based on venous whole blood

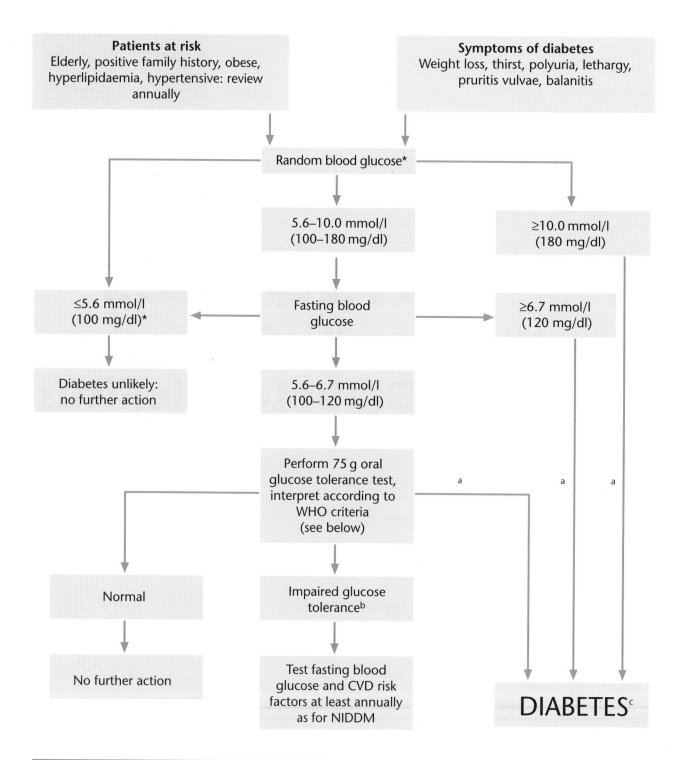

---

[a] In the absence of obvious symptoms, only if value is confirmed at least once

[b] 2 hour value 6.7–9.9 mmol/l (120–179 mg/dl) venous blood; 7.8–11.0 mmol/l (140–199 mg/dl) for capillary blood

[c] 2 hour value ≥10.0 mmol/l (≥180 mg/dl) venous blood; ≥11.1 mmol/l (≥200 mg/dl) for capillary blood

* For random blood glucose, capillary blood will be approximately 1 mmol/l higher. Venous plasma will be 12–14% higher than the quoted whole blood figures

Diabetes: Management of non-insulin dependent diabetes mellitus

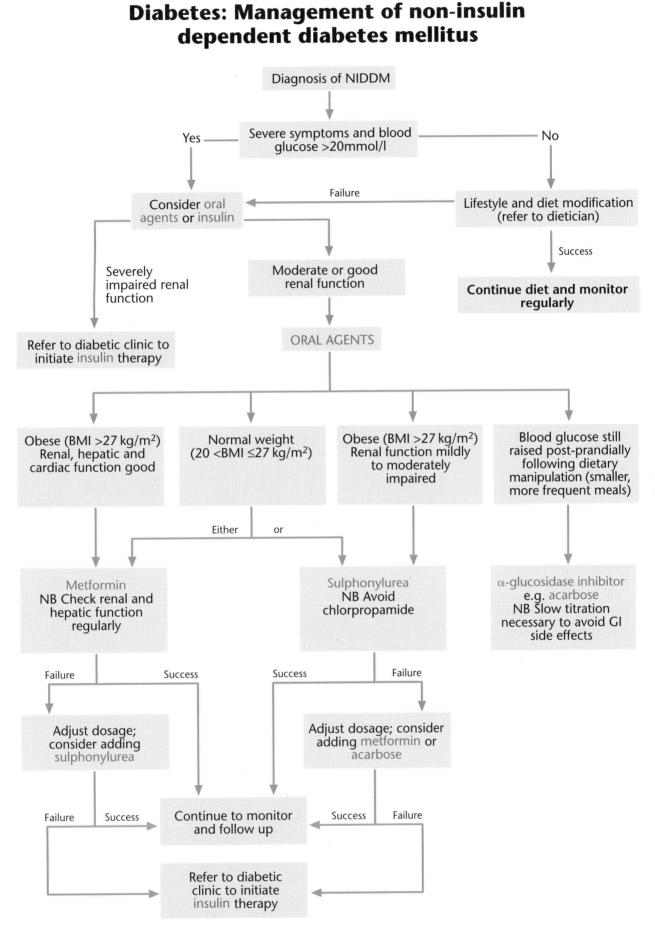

Success: Satisfactory glycaemic control and absence of symptoms
Failure: Poor glycaemic control with or without symptoms persisting after at least 3 months of therapy

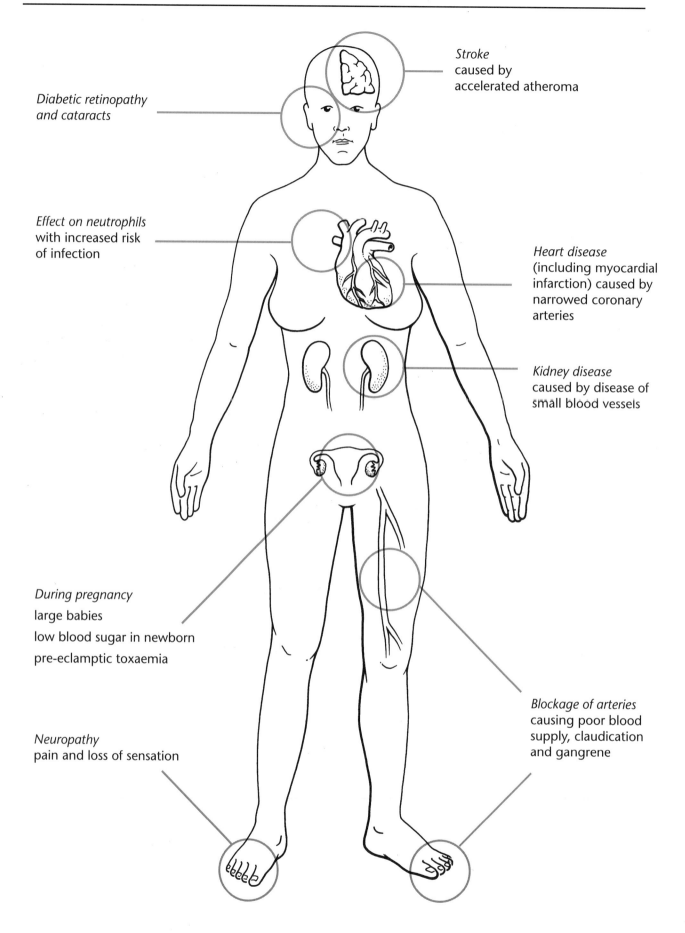

Stroke
caused by
accelerated atheroma

*Diabetic retinopathy
and cataracts*

Effect on neutrophils
with increased risk
of infection

Heart disease
(including myocardial
infarction) caused by
narrowed coronary
arteries

Kidney disease
caused by disease of
small blood vessels

During pregnancy
large babies
low blood sugar in newborn
pre-eclamptic toxaemia

Blockage of arteries
causing poor blood
supply, claudication
and gangrene

Neuropathy
pain and loss of sensation

Figure 7.1   The major complications of diabetes.

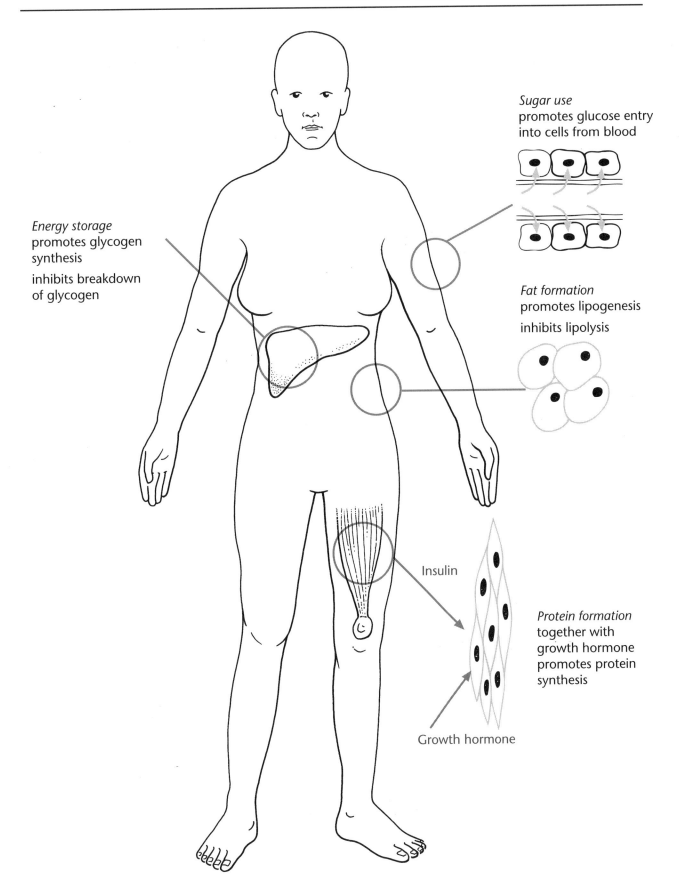

Sugar use
promotes glucose entry
into cells from blood

Fat formation
promotes lipogenesis
inhibits lipolysis

Energy storage
promotes glycogen
synthesis

inhibits breakdown
of glycogen

Insulin

Protein formation
together with
growth hormone
promotes protein
synthesis

Growth hormone

Figure 7.2 Important actions of insulin.

Diabetes references

This guideline is based on:
European NIDDM Policy Group (1993) *A Desk-top Guide to the Management of NIDDM*. International Diabetes Foundation, Brussels, and National Prescribing Centre (1996) Non-insulin dependent diabetes mellitus (part 2). *MeReC Bulletin*: **7**; 30.

Alberti KG and Gries FA (1988) Management of non-insulin-dependent diabetes in Europe: a consensus view. *Diabetic Med*: **5**; 275–81.

American Diabetes Association (1989) Role of cardiovascular risk factors in prevention and treatment of macrovascular disease in diabetes. *Diabetes Care*: **12**; 573–9.

Chalmers I (1992) *Assessing the effects of health technologies, principles, practice, proposals. A paper prepared by the advisory group on Health Technology Assessment for the Director of Research and Development, NHS Management Executive*. Department of Health, London.

Clinical Standards Advisory Group (1994) *Standards of clinical care for people with diabetes*. HMSO, London.

Diabetes Control and Complications Trial Research Group (1993) The effect of intensive treatment of diabetes on the development and progression of long-term complications in insulin-dependent mellitus. *N Engl J Med*: **329**; 977–86.

Greenhalgh PM (1994) Shared care for diabetes: a systematic review. *Royal Coll Gen Pract* (occasional paper 67).

Harris MI (1990) Non-insulin dependent diabetes mellitus in black and white Americans. *Diabetes Metab Rev*: **6**; 71–90.

Harris MI, Klein R, Welborn TA *et al.* (1992) Onset of NIDDM occurs at least 4–7 yrs before clinical diagnosis. *Diabetes Care*: **15**; 815–9.

Javitt JC and Aiello LP (1996) Cost-effectiveness of detecting and treating diabetic retinopathy. *Ann Intern Med*: **124**; 164–9.

Panzram G (1987) Mortality and survival in type 2 (non-insulin dependent) diabetes mellitus *Diabetologia*: **30**; 123–31.

United Kingdom Prospective Diabetes Study (1990) Complications in newly diagnosed type 2 diabetic patients and their association with different clinical and biochemical risk factors. *Diabetes Res*: **13**; 1–11.

United Kingdom Prospective Diabetes Study Group (1996) UKPDS 17: A 9-year update of a randomized, controlled trial on the effect of improved metabolic control on complications in non-insulin dependent diabetes mellitus. *Ann Intern Med*: **124**; 136–45.

8

Duodenal Ulcer

– Suspected or Relapsed

Suspected duodenal ulcer

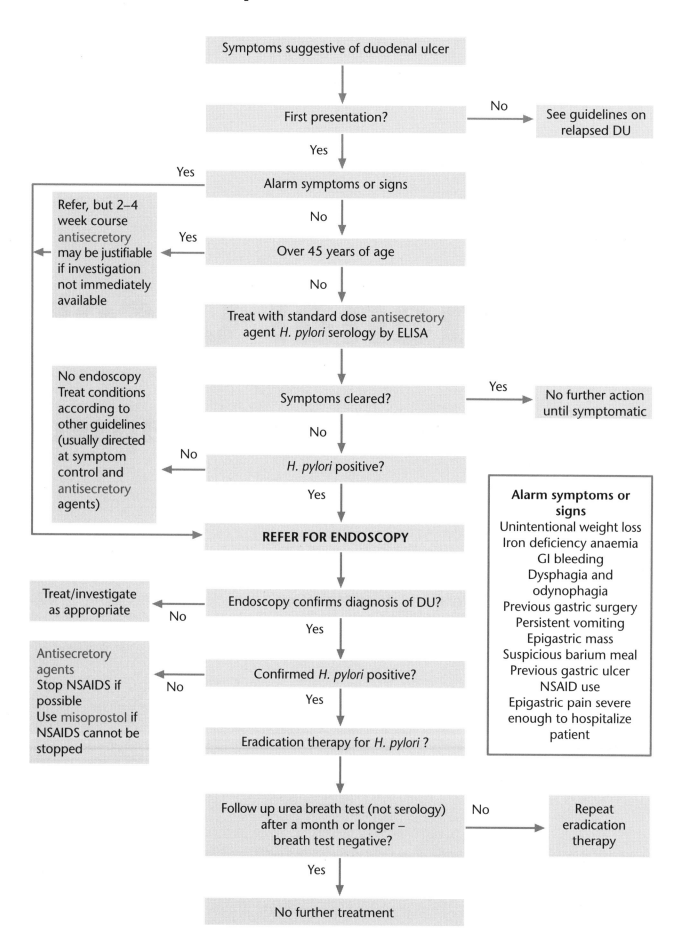

Symptoms suggestive of duodenal ulcer

First presentation? — No → See guidelines on relapsed DU

Yes

Alarm symptoms or signs — Yes → Refer, but 2–4 week course antisecretory may be justifiable if investigation not immediately available

No

Over 45 years of age — Yes →

No

Treat with standard dose antisecretory agent *H. pylori* serology by ELISA

Symptoms cleared? — Yes → No further action until symptomatic

No

H. pylori positive? — No → No endoscopy Treat conditions according to other guidelines (usually directed at symptom control and antisecretory agents)

Yes

REFER FOR ENDOSCOPY

Endoscopy confirms diagnosis of DU? — No → Treat/investigate as appropriate

Yes

Confirmed *H. pylori* positive? — No → Antisecretory agents Stop NSAIDS if possible Use misoprostol if NSAIDS cannot be stopped

Yes

Eradication therapy for *H. pylori* ?

Follow up urea breath test (not serology) after a month or longer – breath test negative? — No → Repeat eradication therapy

Yes

No further treatment

Alarm symptoms or signs
Unintentional weight loss
Iron deficiency anaemia
GI bleeding
Dysphagia and odynophagia
Previous gastric surgery
Persistent vomiting
Epigastric mass
Suspicious barium meal
Previous gastric ulcer
NSAID use
Epigastric pain severe enough to hospitalize patient

Relapsed duodenal ulcer

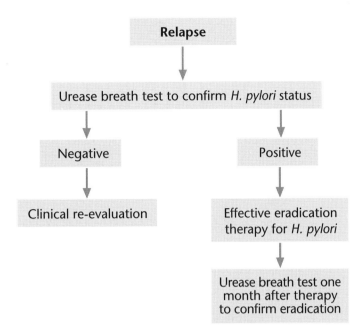

'Best buy' eradication regimens recommended by BSG:

One week triple therapy:
Omeprazole 20 mg b.d. (or lanzoprazole 30 mg b.d.), amoxycillin 500 mg t.d.s. metronidazole 400 mg t.d.s.
Eradication rate 84–90%, well tolerated. Cost: £20.12

Omeprazole 20 mg b.d. (or lanzoprazole 30 mg b.d.), clarithromycin 500 mg b.d. tinidazole 500 mg b.d. (or metronidazole 400 mg b.d.)
Eradication rate around 90%, well tolerated. Cost: £37.02

Omeprazole 20 mg b.d. (or lanzoprazole 30 mg b.d.), amoxycillin 1g b.d. clarithromycin 500 mg b.d.
Eradication rate around 90%, well tolerated. Cost: £42.00 approx.

Traditional two week triple therapy:
Oxytetracycline 500 mg q.d.s., metronidazole 400 mg t.d.s. tripotassium dicitrato bismuthate
Eradication rate 90%, poorly tolerated

HP-ve duodenal ulcer
Antisecretory therapy
Gastroenterological referral if not due to NSAIDS
Stop NSAIDS if possible
Long term treatment with antisecretories or misoprostol may be necessary if NSAIDS are continued

---

Erosive duodenitis
Considered to be part of the spectrum of duodenal ulcer – treat as DU

Patients presenting with complications
(These patients would previously be treated with long term antisecretories to prevent recurrence)
If the urease breath test is negative at follow up, no long term therapy is now recommended
If positive, a further eradication course is indicated

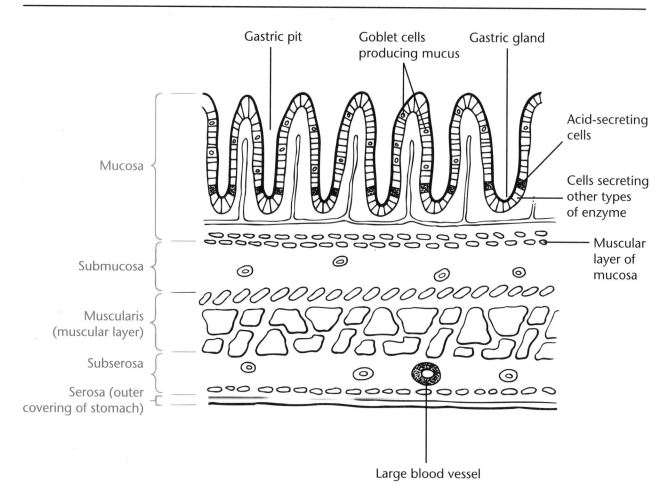

Figure 8.1 Structure of stomach wall.

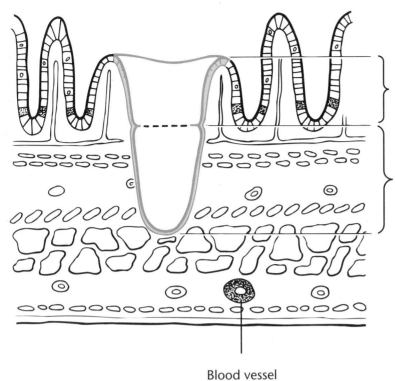

When the damage is this deep it is known as an **erosion**

When the destruction has penetrated the mucosa (and usually into the submucosa and muscularis layers) it is a **true ulcer**

Blood vessel

Figure 8.2   Formation of a true ulcer.

An ulcer can erode the wall of a blood
vessel leading to haemorrhage. It can also
penetrate the outer wall leading to *perforation*,
or cause *scarring* and block the stomach outlet

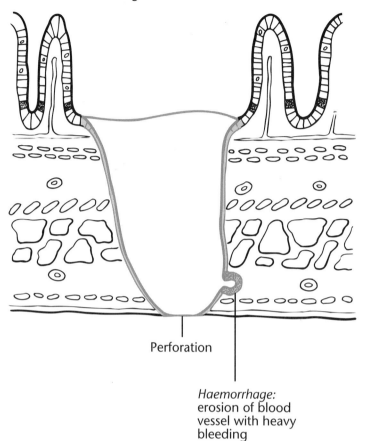

Perforation

Haemorrhage:
erosion of blood
vessel with heavy
bleeding

Figure 8.3   Complications of peptic ulceration.

Suspected and relapsed duodenal ulcer references

This guideline is based on:
British Society of Gastroenterology (1996) *Guidelines in Gastroenterology: 1: Dyspepsia Management Guidelines*. BSG, London.

Adamek RJ, Opferkuch W and Wegener M (1995) Modified short-term triple therapy – ranitidine, clarithromycin, and metronidazole – for cure of *Helicobacter pylori* infection. *Am J Gastroenterol*: **90**; 168–9.

Axon AT, Bell GD, Quine MA *et al.* (1995) Guidelines on the appropriate indications for upper gastrointestinal endoscopy. Working Party of the Joint Committee of the Royal College of Physicians of London, Royal College of Surgeons of England, Royal College of Anaesthetists, Association of Surgeons, the British Society of Gastroenterology and the Thoracic Society of Great Britain. *BMJ*: **310**; 816–17.

De Boer W, Driessen W, Janez A *et al.* (1995) Effect of acid suppression on efficacy of treatment for *Helicobacter pylori* infection. *Lancet*: **345**; 817–20.

Goddard A and Logan R (1995) One-week low-dose triple therapy: new standards for *Helicobacter pylori* treatment. *Eur J Gastroenterol Hepatol*: **7**; 1–3.

Goulston KJ, Dent OF, Mant A *et al.* (1991) Use of H_2 receptor antagonists in patients with dyspepsia and heartburn: a cost comparison. *Med J Aust*: **155**; 20–6.

Hentschel E, Brandstatter G, Dragosics B *et al.* (1993) Effect of ranitidine and amoxycillin plus metronidazole on the eradication of *Helicobacter pylori* and the recurrence of duodenal ulcer. *N Engl J Med*: **328**; 308–12.

Lee A (1991) *Helicobacter pylori*: causal agent in peptic ulcer disease? Working Party Report to the World Congresses of Gastroenterology, Sydney 1990. *J Gastroenterol Hepatol*: **6**; 103–40.

Logan RPH, Gummett PA, Schaufelberger HD *et al.* (1994) Eradication of *Helicobacter pylori* with clarithromycin and omeprazole. *Gut*: **35**; 323–6.

NHS Centre for Reviews and Dissemination (1995) Helicobacter pylori and peptic ulcer. *Effectiveness Matters*: **1**(2).

Savarino V, Mela GS, Zentilin P *et al.* (1993) Acid inhibition and amoxycillin activity against *Helicobacter pylori*. *Am J Gastroenterol*: **88**; 1975–6.

Talley NJ, Colin-Jones D, Koch IK *et al.* (1991) Functional dyspepsia: a classification with guidelines for diagnosis and management. *Gastroenterol Int*: **4**; 145–60.

9

Dyspepsia

Dyspepsia

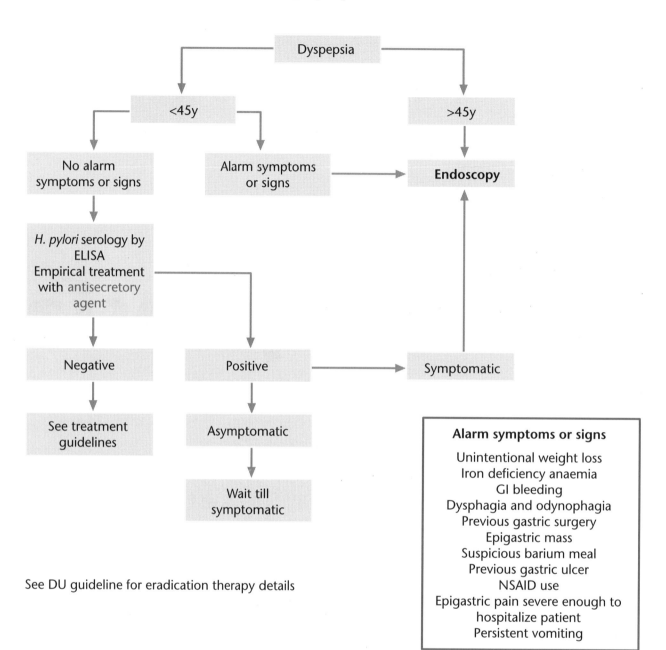

See DU guideline for eradication therapy details

Dyspepsia

Appropriate use of endoscopy

A *Patients with dyspepsia in whom diagnostic endoscopy is appropriate*
1 Any dyspeptic patient with alarm symptoms or signs
2 Any patient over the age of 45 with recent onset dyspepsia
3 Patients under the age of 45 with troublesome dyspepsia who are positive for *H. pylori* on non-invasive testing

B *Patients with dyspepsia in whom endoscopy is inappropriate*
1 Patients known to have duodenal ulcer who have responded symptomatically to treatment
2 Patients under 45 asymptomatic after a single episode of dyspepsia
3 Patients who have recently undergone a satisfactory endoscopy for the same symptoms

Note: Of the small number of patients who develop gastric Ca under the age of 45, the majority are seropositive for *H. pylori*. So these cases too would be diagnosed even in the rare absence of alarm symptoms.

Gastric ulcer

Helicobacter present in 70% – most others due to NSAIDS

Cytological smears, biopsies and urease test taken at endoscopy

HP+ve GU
● Antihelicobacter therapy as for duodenal ulcer *followed by antisecretory therapy for two months* (no evidence that GUs heal as quickly after *H. pylori* eradication alone)
● Long term treatment with misoprostol considered in patients with proven ulcer who must take an NSAID

HP–ve GU
● Standard antisecretory therapy for two months
● Stop NSAIDS if possible. Omeprazole more effective than H2 antagonist if NSAID continued
● Long term treatment with misoprostol considered if proven ulcer, needing to continue with NSAID

Follow up
Repeat endoscopy is essential until complete epithelialisation. If ulcer unhealed for six months, surgery should be considered

Dyspepsia references

This guideline is based on:
British Society of Gastroenterology (1996) *Guidelines in Gastroenterology: 1: Dyspepsia Management Guidelines.* BSG, London. Copies can be obtained from British Society of Gastroenterology, 3 St Andrews Place, Regent's Park, London NW1 4LB, price £4.

Axon AT, Bell GD, Quine MA *et al.* (1995) Guidelines on the appropriate indications for upper GI endoscopy. *BMJ*: **310**; 816–17.

Bytzer P, Hansen JM, de Muckadell OBS (1994) Empirical H2 blocker therapy or prompt endoscopy in management of dyspepsia. *Lancet*: **343**; 811–16.

Chiba N, Rao BV, Rademaker JW *et al.* (1992) Meta-analysis of the efficacy of antibiotic therapy in eradicating Helicobacter pylori. *Am J Gastroent*: **87**; 1716–27.

Forman D (1995) The prevalence of Helicobacter pylori in gastric cancer. *Aliment Pharmacol Ther*: **9** (Suppl. 2); 71–6.

Gough AL, Long RG, Cooper BT *et al.* (1996) Lansoprazole versus ranitidine in the maintenance treatment of reflux oesophagitis. *Aliment Pharmacol Ther*: **10**; 529–39.

Jones R (1988) What happens to patients with non-ulcer dyspepsia after endoscopy? *Practitioner*: **232**; 75–8.

Mendall MA, Goggin PM, Marrero JM *et al.* (1992) Helicobacter screening prior to endoscopy. *Eur J Gastroent Hepat*: **4**; 713–17.

NHS Centre for Reviews and Dissemination (1995) Helicobacter pylori and peptic ulcer. *Effectiveness Matters*: **1**(2).

Patel P, Khulusi S, Mendall MA *et al.* (1995) Prospective screening of dyspeptic patients by Helicobacter pylori serology. *Lancet*: **346**; 1315–18.

Sonneneberg A and Townsend WF (1995) Costs of duodenal ulcer therapy with antibiotics. *Archives of Int Med*: **155**; 922–8.

Walsh JH and Peterson WL (1995) The treatment of Helicobacter pylori infection in the management of peptic ulcer disease. *N Engl J Med*: **333**; 984–91.

Waugh NR (1996) Cost effectiveness of screening for and eradication of Helicobacter pylori in young patients with dyspepsia. Cost of eradication treatment may have been overestimated. *BMJ*: **313**; 622.

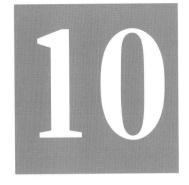

Eczema

| | Eczema – hands and feet | | Contact dermatitis | Seborrhoeic dermatitis | Discoid eczema | Atopic eczema | Stasis eczema |
Types	Chronic	Acute pompholyx					
Diagnostic characteristics	Excluding psoriasis, fungus; Palms and soles often prominently involved; Dry, scaly or fissured areas	Itchy or painful blisters on palms and fingers, toes and soles	Itchy, scaly skin; Sites of contact with allergens or irritants; Often occupational	Dull red patches, greasy and/or scaly; On scalp and face	Round or oval patches of red, scaly or weeping skin	Itchy red and dry skin; Often starts in childhood	Elderly patients; Varicose veins; Oedema
First-line treatments	Moderately potent or potent topical corticosteroid and emollients	Potassium permanganate (0.1%); Potent topical corticosteroid and emollient; Oral corticosteroids may be required	Treat acute episodes with potent topical corticosteroid; Avoidance measures	'Medicated' shampoo or ketoconazole shampoo/cream; Salicylic acid ointment or topical corticosteroid scalp preparation; Imidazole/hydrocortisone combination	Moderately potent or potent corticosteroid	Topical corticosteroid (potency dependent on site) and emollients; Mild topical corticosteroids should be used on the face and flexures – for trunk and limbs use two-step approach (see box below); Children (see box below); Avoid aggravating factors	Moderately potent or potent topical corticosteroid; Compression stockings if circulation is adequate; Titrate topical corticosteroid to lowest effective dose
Duration of treatment	Chronic administration at lowest dose to control symptoms	14 days initially and reassess; Secondary bacterial infection should be treated with flucloxacillin	Review after one week, and reduce to moderately potent topical corticosteroids for three to four weeks; Regular application of emollients	Should respond within a few days although lesions usually recur	Lesions settle quickly but new ones will usually continue to occur	To control acute symptoms; Persistent lichenified areas may require treatment over a long period	14 days with moderate/potent topical corticosteroid; Maintenance therapy with 1% hydrocortisone or equivalent
Referral criteria	If possibility of contact dermatitis	Repeated episodes	For patch testing	Failure to respond to first-line therapy	Failure to control	Failure of first-line therapy; Suspected contact allergy; Suspected secondary infection with herpes simplex; Worsening of eczema	For Doppler scanning if peripheral circulation is suspect; For patch testing where condition persists
Management issues	Advise on care of hands; Refer for patch testing; Refer for hospital treatment e.g. PUVA	Advise on care of hands; Refer for patch testing if recurrent	May become chronic: refer for patch testing; Acute exacerbations: Potent topical corticosteroids/oral corticosteroids if necessary	Severe seborrhoeic dermatitis may indicate HIV infection	Often infected, use topical corticosteroid/anti-infective combination; Often a chronic problem	Often chronic, reduce topical corticosteroid to lowest dose to maintain symptom control. Watch for secondary infection; Offer career advice	Doppler scan to establish if circulation is adequate to permit use of compression stockings

Two-step approach

A two-step therapeutic approach is recommended. Use a mild/moderate potency corticosteroid for long-term maintenance treatment, but a potent topical corticosteroid for short-term use (five to seven days) in an acute flare

Topical steroids in children

In infants and young children, use a mild topical steroid. Some moderately potent corticosteroids may be no more likely to cause unwanted side-effects than hydrocortisone (e.g. 0.05% clobetasone butyrate 0.05% alclometasone dipropionate). Consider referring for specialist supervision if moderately potent corticosteroids are required for prolonged periods.
Children requiring potent or very potent topical corticosteroids should be referred for specialist supervision

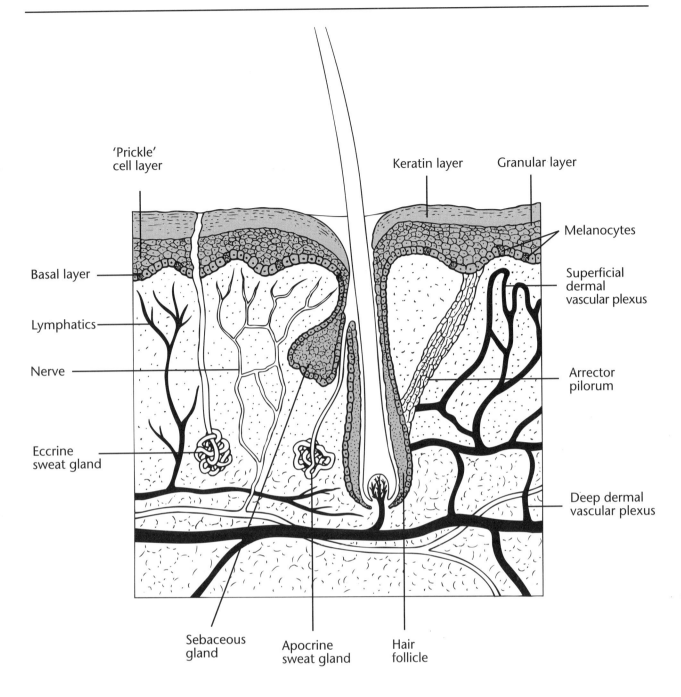

'Prickle' cell layer

Keratin layer

Granular layer

Melanocytes

Basal layer

Lymphatics

Nerve

Superficial dermal vascular plexus

Arrector pilorum

Eccrine sweat gland

Deep dermal vascular plexus

Sebaceous gland

Apocrine sweat gland

Hair follicle

Figure 10.1 Normal epidermis.

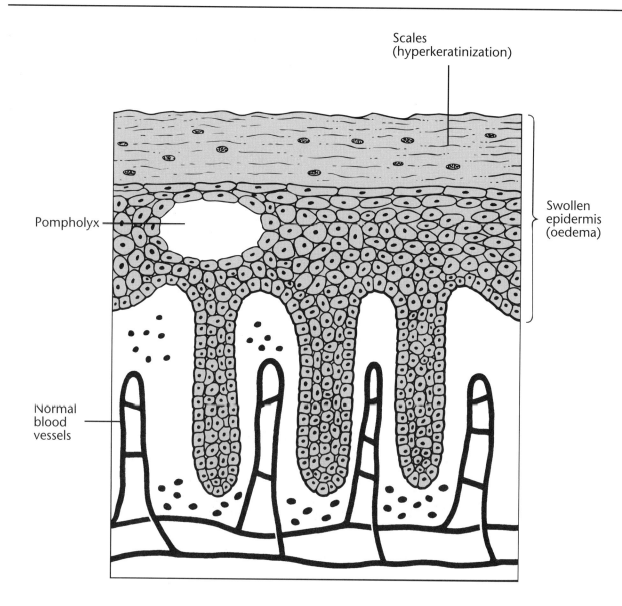

Scales
(hyperkeratinization)

Swollen
epidermis
(oedema)

Pompholyx

Normal
blood
vessels

Figure 10.2 Eczema.

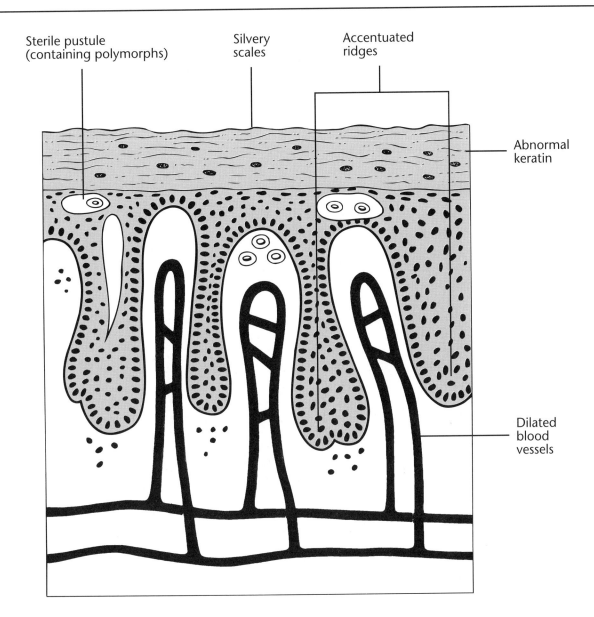

Sterile pustule
(containing polymorphs)

Silvery
scales

Accentuated
ridges

Abnormal
keratin

Dilated
blood
vessels

Figure 10.3 Psoriasis.

Eczema references

This guideline is based on:
Action Plans produced from a workshop on the management of eczema in general practice, May 1994. Full guidelines are published by Colwood Medical Publications.

Arshad SH, Matthews S, Gant C *et al.* (1992) Effect of allergen avoidance on allergic disorders in infancy. *Lancet*: **339**; 1493–7.

Bos JD, Kapsenberg ML and Sillevis Smitt JH (1994) Pathogenesis of atopic eczema. *Lancet*: **343**; 1338–41.

Finlay AY and Khan GK (1994) Dermatology life quality index (D1–Q1): a simple practical measure for routine clinical use. *Clin Exp Dermatol*: **19**; 210–16.

Golding J and Peters TJ (1987) The epidemiology of childhood eczema. *Paediatr Perinatal Epidemiol*: **1**; 67–9.

Howell JB (1976) Eye diseases induced by topically applied steroids. *Arch Dermatol*: **112**; 1529–30.

Long CC, Collard R, Funnel CM *et al.* (1993) What do members of the National Eczema Society really want? *Clin Exp Dermatol*: **18**(6); 516–22.

Long CC and Finlay AY (1991) The finger tip unit – a new practical measure. *Clin Exp Dermatol*: **16**; 444–7.

Sheehan MP, Rustin MHA, Atherton DJ *et al.* (1992) Efficacy of traditional Chinese herbal therapy in adult atopic dermatitis: results of a double-blind placebo-controlled study. *Lancet*: **340**; 13–7.

Stewart JCM, Morse PF, Moss M *et al.* (1991) Treatment of severe and moderately severe atopic dermatitis with evening primrose oil (Epogam); a multi-centre study. *J Nutr Med*: **2**; 9–15.

Tan BB, Weald D, Strickland I *et al.* (1996) Double-blind controlled trial of effect of house dust-mite allergen avoidance on atopic dermatitis. *Lancet*: **347**; 15–18.

Williams HC (1992) Is the prevalence of atopic eczema increasing? *Clin Exp Dermatol*: **17**; 385–91.

Williams HC (1995) Atopic eczema (editorial). *BMJ*: **311**; 1241–2.

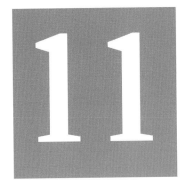

Haematuria

Microscopic

>40 years

Exclude tumours

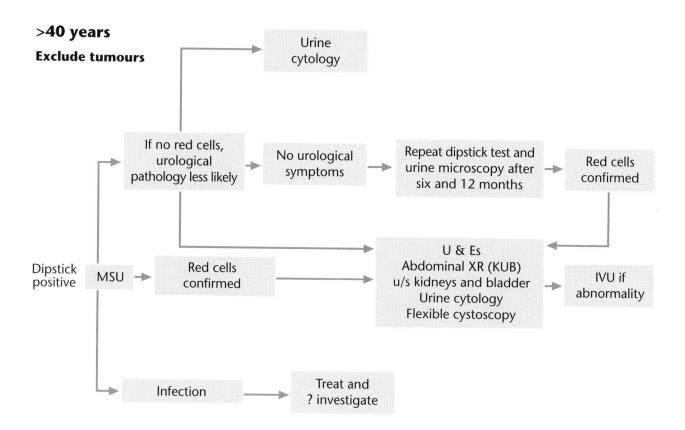

<40 years

Exclude stones, congenital abnormalities and intrinsic renal disease

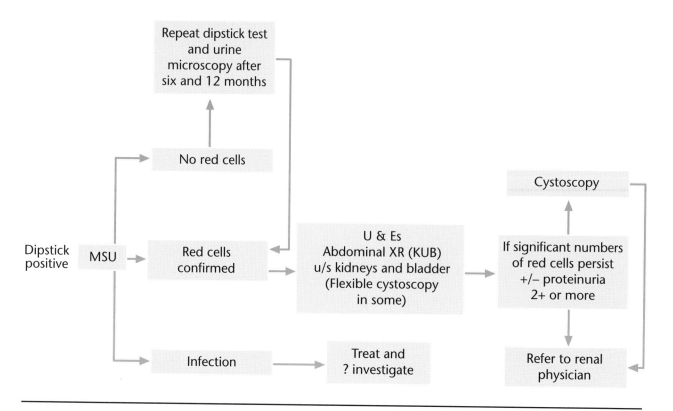

Macroscopic

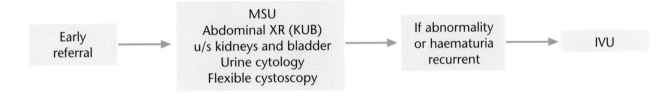

Early referral → MSU / Abdominal XR (KUB) / u/s kidneys and bladder / Urine cytology / Flexible cystoscopy → If abnormality or haematuria recurrent → IVU

Haematuria references

No national guidelines exist at the time of going to print. This guideline was kindly developed by Mr Philip Britton, Consultant Urological Surgeon, St Richard's Hospital, Chichester.

Abdurrahman MB, Kambal AM, Kurbaan K M *et al.* (1986) Diagnostic value of phase contrast microscopy in haematuria. *Brit J Urol*: **58**(2); 211–17.

Arm JP, Peile EB, Rainford DJ *et al.* (1986) Significance of dipstick haematuria. 1. Correlation with microscopy of the urine. *Brit J Urol*: **58**(2); 211–17.

Banks RA and Stower M (1989) Investigation of haematuria in adults. *Brit J Hosp Med*: **41**(5); 476–80 [Review].

Hofmann W, Regenbogen C, Edel H *et al.* (1994) Diagnostic strategies in urinalysis. *Kidney International* (Supplement): **47**; S111–4 Nov.

Janssens PM (1994) New markets for analyzing the cause of hematuria. *Kidney International* (Supplement): **47**; S115–6.

Jones DJ, Langstaff R J, Holt SD *et al.* (1988) The value of cystourethroscopy in the investigation of microscopic haematuria in adult males under 40 years. A prospective study of 100 patients. *Brit J Urol*: **62**(6); 541–5.

Lynch TH, Waymont B, Dunn JA *et al.* (1994) Rapid diagnostic service for patients with haematuria. *Brit J Urol*: **73**(2); 147–51.

Marazzi P and Gabriel R (1994) The haematuria clinic. *BMJ*: **308**; 356 [editorial].

Ng RC and Seto DS (1984) Hematuria. A suggested workup strategy. *Postgrad Med*: **75**(1); 139–44.

Schroder FH (1994) Microscopic haematuria. *BMJ*: **309**; 70–2 [editorial].

White RH (1994) Haematuria clinics. Cystoscopy of little value in children (letter; comment). *BMJ*: **308**; 788.

Hayfever

Hayfever

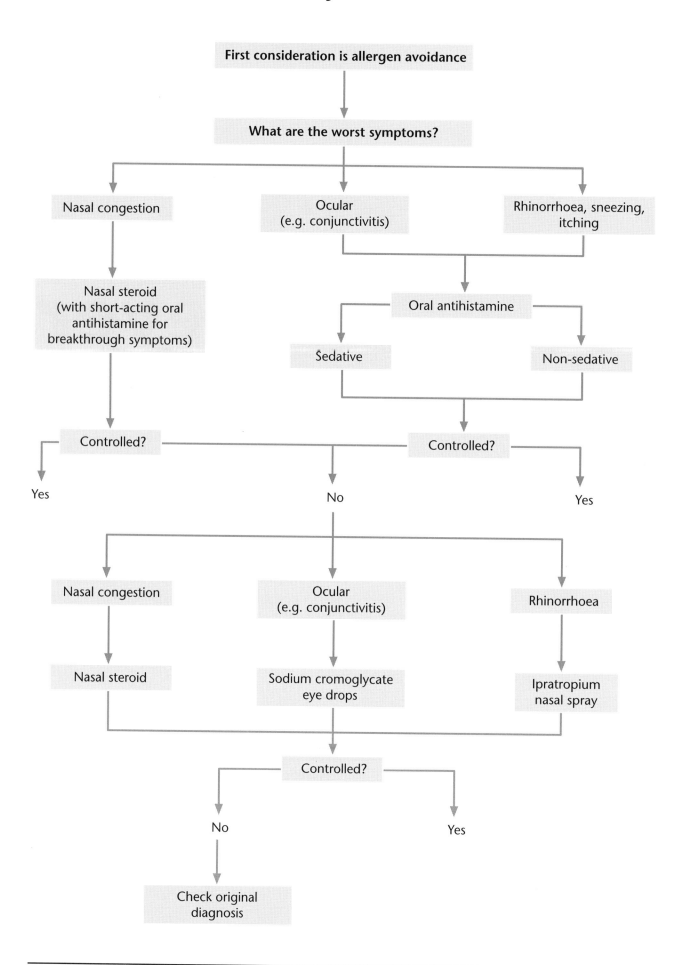

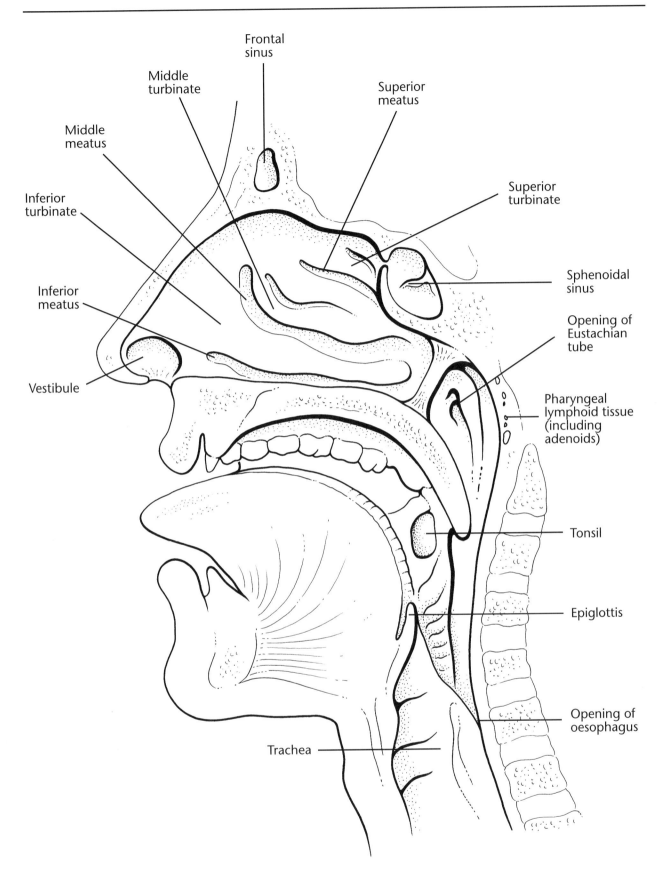

Frontal
sinus

Middle
turbinate

Superior
meatus

Middle
meatus

Superior
turbinate

Inferior
turbinate

Sphenoidal
sinus

Inferior
meatus

Opening of
Eustachian
tube

Vestibule

Pharyngeal
lymphoid tissue
(including
adenoids)

Tonsil

Epiglottis

Opening of
oesophagus

Trachea

Figure 12.1 Anatomy of oral and nasal cavities.

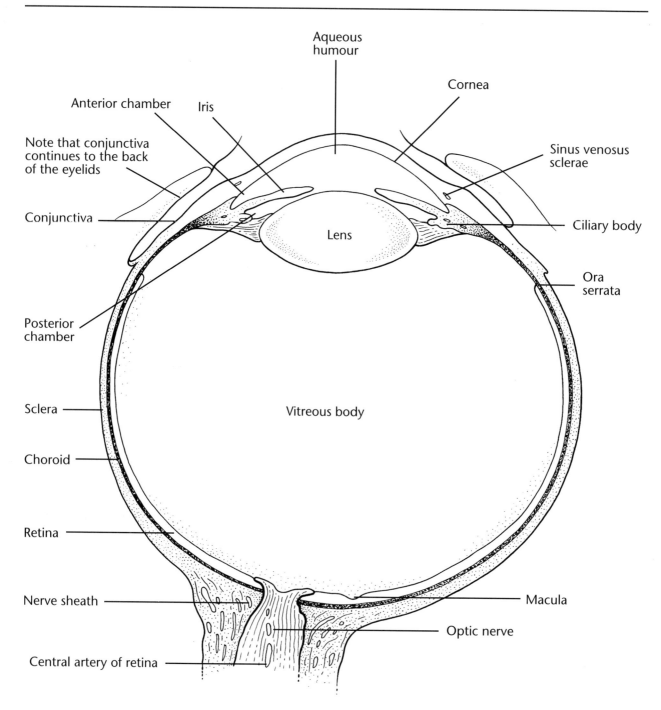

Figure 12.2 Structure of the eye.

Hayfever references

This guideline is adapted from:
The Medical Resource Centre (Liverpool) (1995) Hayfever. *MeReC Bulletin*: **6**(4).

Anon (1993) Terfenadine and astemizole: safe in normal use but precautions required to avoid arrhythmias. *Drugs Therap Perspect*: **2**; 12–13.

Anon (1992) Ventricular arrhythmias due to terfenadine and astemizole. *Current Problems*: No. **35**; 1.

Black MJ and Remsen KA (1980) Rhinitis medicamentosa. *Can Med Assoc J*: **122**; 881–4.

CSM Update (1986) Desensitising vaccines. *Br Med J*: **293**; 948.

Delafuente JC, Davis TA and Davis JA (1989) Pharmacotherapy of allergic rhinitis. *Clin Pharm*: **8**; 474–85.

Estelle F, Simons R and Simons KJ (1989) Optimum pharmacological management of chronic rhinitis. *Drugs*: **38**; 313–31.

Fry J (1987) *Common Diseases. Their Nature, Incidence and Care* (4th edn). MTP Press Ltd, 134–8.

Ross AM and Fleming DM (1994) Incidence of allergic rhinitis in general practice, 1981–92. *BMJ*: **308**; 897–900.

Stafford CT (1987) Allergic rhinitis – a useful guide to diagnosis and treatment. *Postgrad Med*: **81**; 147–57.

Strachan DP, Taylor EM and Carpenter RG (1996) Family structure, neonatal infection and hay fever in adolescence. *Arch Dis Child*: **74**(5); 422–6.

Varney VA, Gaga M, Frew AJ *et al.* (1991) Usefulness of immunotherapy in patients with severe summer hayfever uncontrolled by antiallergic drugs. *Br Med J*: **302**; 265–9.

Wood SF (1990) Rhinitis. *Presc J*: **30**; 197–203.

Headache

Headache

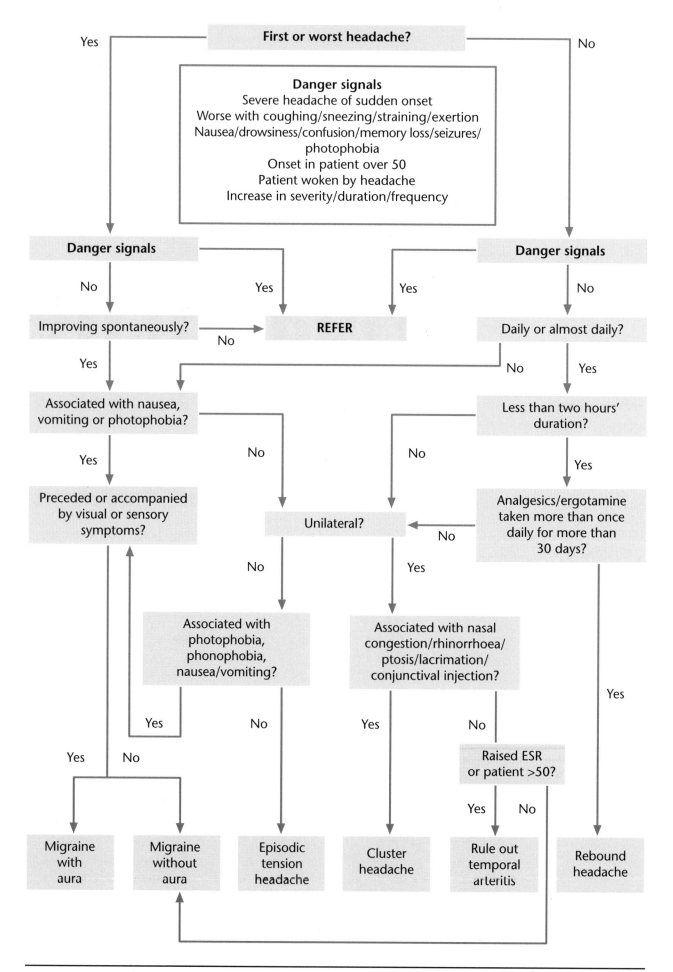

First or worst headache?

Yes — No

Danger signals
Severe headache of sudden onset
Worse with coughing/sneezing/straining/exertion
Nausea/drowsiness/confusion/memory loss/seizures/
photophobia
Onset in patient over 50
Patient woken by headache
Increase in severity/duration/frequency

Danger signals — **Danger signals**

No — Yes — Yes — No

Improving spontaneously? — **REFER** — Daily or almost daily?

No

Yes — No — Yes

Associated with nausea, vomiting or photophobia? — Less than two hours' duration?

Yes — No — No — Yes

Preceded or accompanied by visual or sensory symptoms? — Unilateral? — Analgesics/ergotamine taken more than once daily for more than 30 days?

No — Yes — No

Associated with photophobia, phonophobia, nausea/vomiting? — Associated with nasal congestion/rhinorrhoea/ptosis/lacrimation/conjunctival injection?

Yes — No — Yes — No — Yes

Raised ESR or patient >50?

Yes — No

Yes — No

Migraine with aura — Migraine without aura — Episodic tension headache — Cluster headache — Rule out temporal arteritis — Rebound headache

Headache references

This guideline is based on:
The International Headache Society Classification. This algorithm is based on one published by Glaxo in *Managing Headache – A Guide to Differential Diagnosis* and produced by Synergy Medical Education.

Akpunonu BE, Mutgi AB, Federman DJ *et al.* (1995) Subcutaneous sumatriptan for treatment of acute migraine in patients admitted to the emergency department: a multicenter study. *Annals Emerg Med*: **25**(4); 464–9.

Anonymous (1988) Classification and diagnostic criteria for headache disorders, cranial neuralgias and facial pain. Headache Classification Committee of the International Headache Society. *Cephalalgia*: **8**(Suppl. 7); 1–96.

Cady RK, Rubino J, Crummett D *et al.* (1994) Oral sumatriptan in the treatment of recurrent headache. *Arch Fam Med*: **3**(9); 766–72.

Manzoni GC, Granella F, Sandrini G *et al.* (1995) Classification of chronic daily headache by International Headache Society criteria: limits and new proposals. *Cephalalgia*: **15**(1); 37–43.

Marcus DA, Nash JM, Turk DC (1994) Diagnosing recurring headaches: IHS criteria and beyond. *Headache*: **34**(6); 329–36.

Nappi G, Agnoli A, Manzoni GC *et al.* (1989) Classification and diagnostic criteria for primary headache disorders (AdHoc Committee IHS, 1988). *Fun Neurol*: **4**(1); 65–71.

Olesen J and Lipton RB (1994) Migraine classification and diagnosis. International Headache Society criteria. [Review] *Neurol*: **44**(Suppl. 4); S6–10.

Oleson J (1995) Analgesic headache: a common, treatable condition that deserves more attention. *BMJ*: **310**; 479–80.

Pini LA, Sternieri E, Fabbri L *et al.* (1995) High efficacy and low frequency of headache recurrence after oral sumatriptan. The Oral Sumatriptan Italian Study Group. *J Int Med Res*: **23**(2); 96–105.

Rasmussen BK, Jensen R and Olesen J (1991) A population-based analysis of the diagnostic criteria of the International Headache Society. *Cephalalgia*: **11**(3); 129–34.

Russell MB, Rasmussen BK, Brennum J *et al.* (1992) Presentation of a new instrument: the diagnostic headache diary. *Cephalalgia*: **12**(6); 369–74.

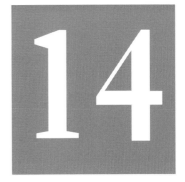

Heart Failure

Heart failure: new patients

Visit one

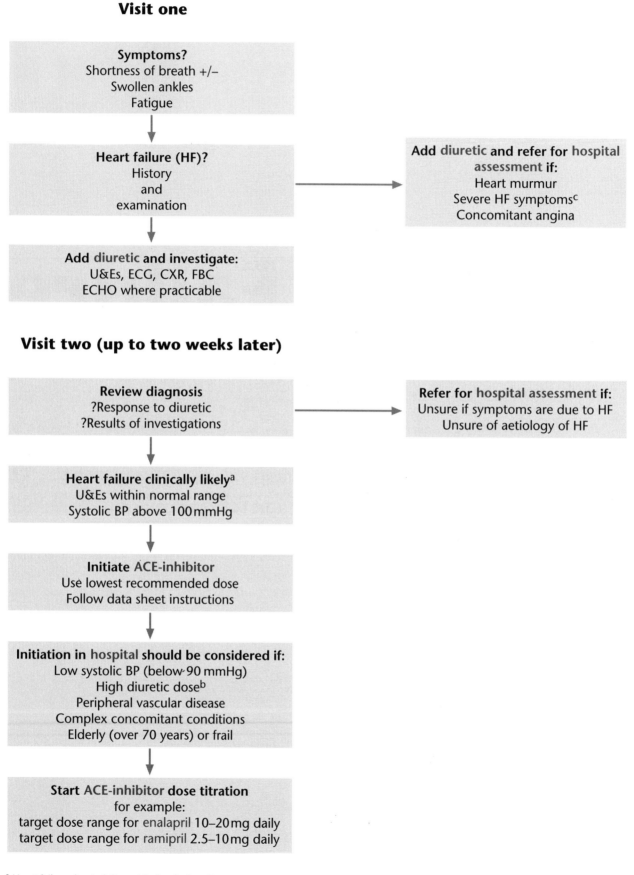

Symptoms?
Shortness of breath +/–
Swollen ankles
Fatigue

↓

Heart failure (HF)?
History
and
examination

Add diuretic and refer for hospital assessment if:
Heart murmur
Severe HF symptoms[c]
Concomitant angina

↓

Add diuretic and investigate:
U&Es, ECG, CXR, FBC
ECHO where practicable

Visit two (up to two weeks later)

Review diagnosis
?Response to diuretic
?Results of investigations

Refer for hospital assessment if:
Unsure if symptoms are due to HF
Unsure of aetiology of HF

↓

Heart failure clinically likely[a]
U&Es within normal range
Systolic BP above 100 mmHg

↓

Initiate ACE-inhibitor
Use lowest recommended dose
Follow data sheet instructions

↓

Initiation in hospital should be considered if:
Low systolic BP (below 90 mmHg)
High diuretic dose[b]
Peripheral vascular disease
Complex concomitant conditions
Elderly (over 70 years) or frail

↓

Start ACE-inhibitor dose titration
for example:
target dose range for enalapril 10–20 mg daily
target dose range for ramipril 2.5–10 mg daily

[a] Heart failure due to left ventricular dysfunction
[b] Patients with hypovolaemia or hyponatraemia may be at higher risk of developing first-dose hypotension
[c] Severe heart failure: treatment with ACE-inhibitors should always be initiated in hospital under close medical supervision

Heart failure: existing patients

Visit one

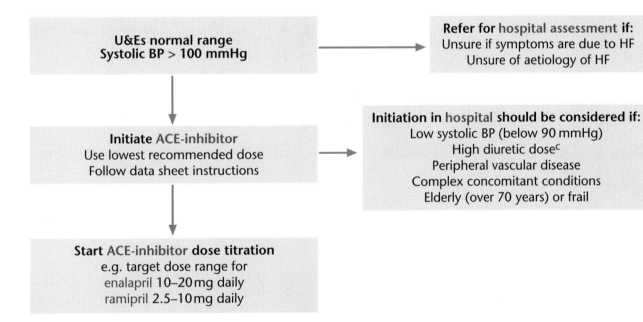

Review diagnosis
History
and
examination

↓

Heart failure confirmed[a]
Obtain U&Es
Review diuretic dose
(Reduce where appropriate)

→

Refer for hospital assessment if:
Heart murmur
Severe HF symptoms[b]
Concomitant angina
Unsure of diagnosis

Visit two (up to two weeks later)

U&Es normal range
Systolic BP > 100 mmHg

→

Refer for hospital assessment if:
Unsure if symptoms are due to HF
Unsure of aetiology of HF

↓

Initiate ACE-inhibitor
Use lowest recommended dose
Follow data sheet instructions

→

Initiation in hospital should be considered if:
Low systolic BP (below 90 mmHg)
High diuretic dose[c]
Peripheral vascular disease
Complex concomitant conditions
Elderly (over 70 years) or frail

↓

Start ACE-inhibitor dose titration
e.g. target dose range for
enalapril 10–20 mg daily
ramipril 2.5–10 mg daily

[a] Heart failure due to left ventricular dysfunction
[b] Severe heart failure: treatment with ACE-inhibitors should always be initiated in hospital under close medical supervision
[c] Patients with hypovolaemia or hyponatraemia may be at higher risk of developing first-dose hypotension

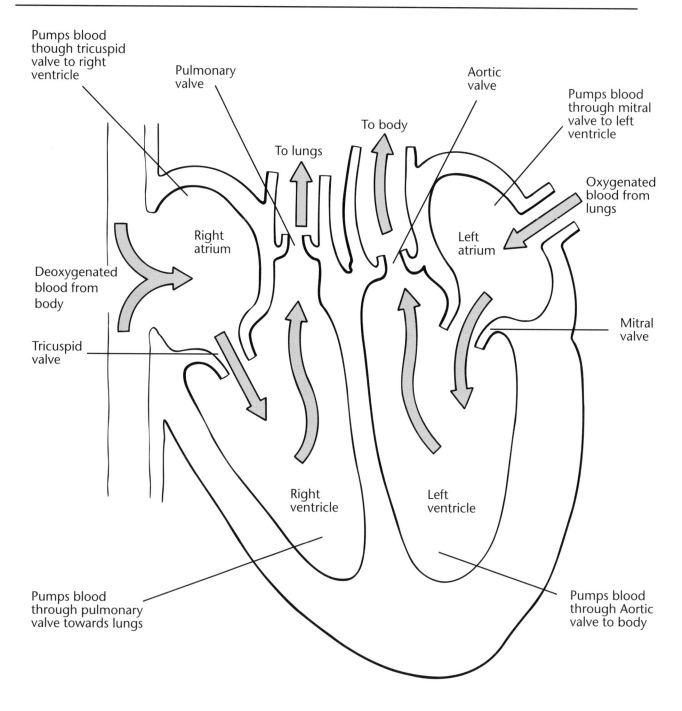

Pumps blood though tricuspid valve to right ventricle

Pulmonary valve

Aortic valve

Pumps blood through mitral valve to left ventricle

To lungs

To body

Right atrium

Left atrium

Oxygenated blood from lungs

Deoxygenated blood from body

Tricuspid valve

Mitral valve

Right ventricle

Left ventricle

Pumps blood through pulmonary valve towards lungs

Pumps blood through Aortic valve to body

Figure 14.1 Blood flow through normal heart.

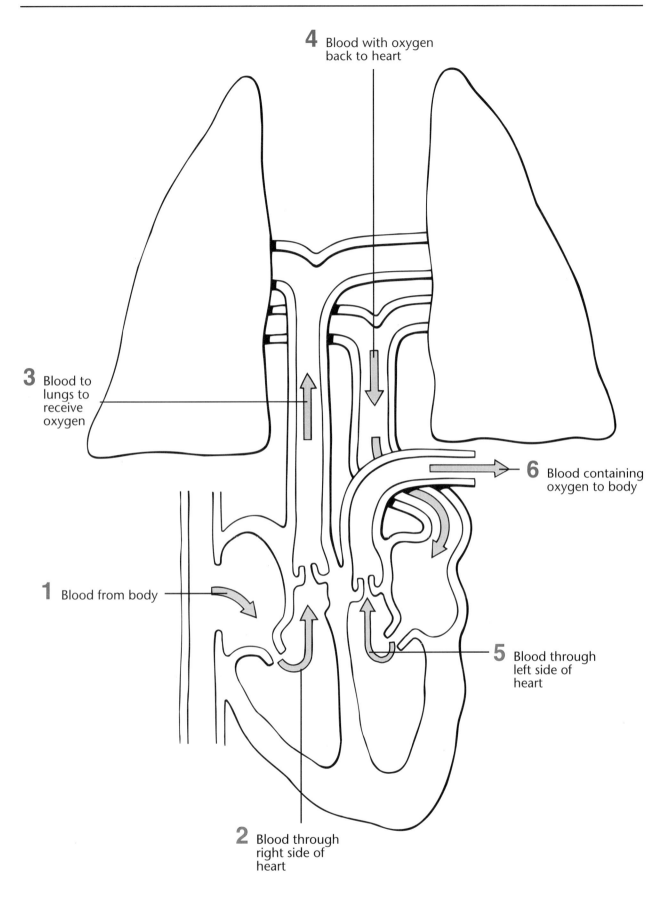

4 Blood with oxygen back to heart

3 Blood to lungs to receive oxygen

6 Blood containing oxygen to body

1 Blood from body

5 Blood through left side of heart

2 Blood through right side of heart

Figure 14.2 Blood flow through normal heart and lungs.

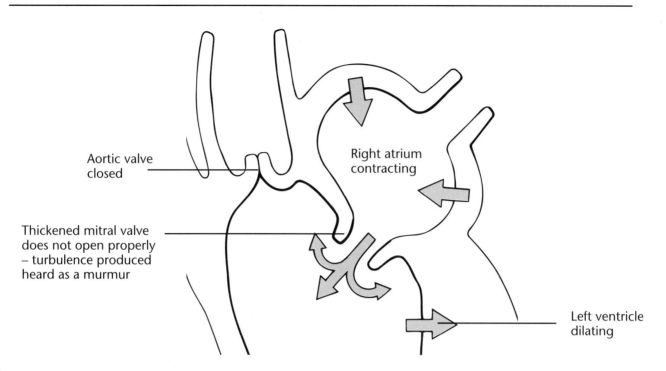

Aortic valve
closed

Right atrium
contracting

Thickened mitral valve
does not open properly
– turbulence produced
heard as a murmur

Left ventricle
dilating

Figure 14.3   Heart valve disease: mitral stenosis.

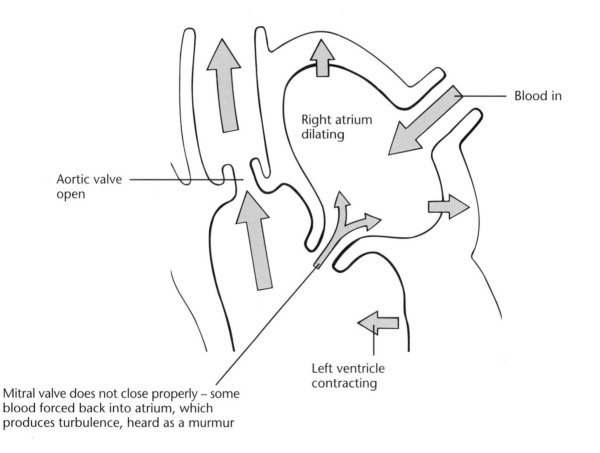

Blood in

Right atrium
dilating

Aortic valve
open

Left ventricle
contracting

Mitral valve does not close properly – some
blood forced back into atrium, which
produces turbulence, heard as a murmur

Figure 14.4   Heart valve disease: mitral incompetence.

Heart failure references

This guideline is based on:
The Heart Failure Task Force guidelines in identifying and treating new sufferers from heart failure in: *Heart Failure: A Change for the Better. Management Protocol (1992).*

Acute Infarction Ramipril Efficacy (AIRE) Study Investigators (1993) Effect of ramipril on mortality and morbidity of survivors of acute myocardial infarction with clinical evidence of heart failure. *Lancet*: **342**; 821–8.

Clark AL and Coats AJS (1995) Severity of heart failure and dosage of angiotensin converting enzyme inhibitors. *BMJ*: **310**; 973–4.

Dickstein K, Chang P, Willenheimer R *et al.* (1995) Comparison of the effects of losartan and enalapril on clinical status and exercise performance in patients with moderate or severe chronic heart failure. *Am Coll Cardiol*: **26**(2); 438–45.

Gruppo Italiano per la Studio della Sopravvivenza nell-Infarto Miocardico (1994) *GISSI-3*: effects of Lisinopril and transdermal glyceryl trinitrate singly and together on 6-week mortality and ventricular function after acute myocardial infarction. *Lancet*: **343**; 1115–22.

Kleber FX, Niemöller L and Doering W (1992) Impact of converting enzyme inhibition on progression of chronic heart failure: Munich mild heart failure trial. *Br Heart J*: **67**; 289–96.

McMurray J, Hart W and Rhodes G (1993) An evaluation of the cost of heart failure to the National Health Service in the UK. *Br Med Econ*: **6**; 99–110.

Northridge D (1996) Frusemide or nitrates for acute heart failure? *Lancet*: **347**; 667–8.

Packer M, Gheorghiade M, Young JB *et al.* (1993) For the RADIANCE study. Withdrawal of digoxin from patients with chronic heart failure treated with angiotensin-converting-enzyme inhibitors. *N Engl J Med*: **329**; 1–7.

Rowe PM (1994) Guidelines for management of heart failure. *Lancet*: **344**; 123.

The SOLVD Investigators (1991) Effect of enalapril on survival in patients with reduced left ventricular ejection fractions and congestive heart failure. *N Engl J Med*: **325**; 293–301.

The SOLVD Investigators (1992) Effect of enalapril on mortality and the development of heart failure in asymptomatic patients with reduced left ventricular ejection fraction. *N Engl J Med*: **327**; 685–91.

Yusuf S, Pepine CJ, Garces C *et al.* (1992) Effect of enalapril on myocardial infarction and unstable angina in patients with low ejection fractions. *Lancet*: **340**; 1173–8.

Hip and Knee Replacement – GP Referral

Hip and knee replacement

Appropriateness for GP referral and case selection for hip or knee replacement

The Delphi method was used to create these guidelines. The algorithms uses a scoring system based on an expert panel's pooled decisions, based on given clinical scenarios.

Appropriateness for referral

Extremely vigorous activity is contraindicated after joint replacement, prosthesis failure rates rise after 10 years and reoperation is technically difficult. Hence, particularly in people under 60 years of age without considerably impaired function, it is prudent to defer surgery or consider alternative procedures such as high tibial osteotomy or femoral osteotomy whenever feasible.

Functional Class and summary of guidelines

(American College of Rheumatology definitions of functional class in italics)

Class I
Complete functional capacity with ability to carry on all usual duties without handicaps

Class II
Functional capacity adequate to conduct normal activities despite handicap of discomfort or limited mobility of one or more joints
- When pain is mild or osteotomy is an option, joint replacement is deemed inappropriate for patients in functional Class II (Scores 1.00 and 1.33 respectively)
- Even among those who cannot have an osteotomy and who have moderate pain, the appropriateness of joint replacement is uncertain and highly dependent on case specific judgements, unless patients are older and have a good chance of prosthesis survival

Class III
Functional capacity adequate to perform only few or none of the duties of usual occupation or of self care
- Again, osteotomy is deemed preferable to arthroplasty whenever possible in patients younger than 60
- For those not able to undergo osteotomy, the need for pain relief must be weighed against chances of long term prosthesis survival
- If pain is mild, surgery should be viewed cautiously unless there is a very good chance of long term prosthesis survival
- Among older patients (>60), moderate and severe pain are strong indications for joint replacement when coupled with impaired activities of daily living as is usual in this functional class

Class IV
Largely or wholly incapacitated with a patient bedridden or confined to wheelchair, permitting little or no self care
- Patients are bedridden or confined to a wheelchair, or both, hence pain on activity is not a factor
- Patients with severe rest pain are potentially appropriate regardless of other factors, as joint replacement may be the only option to relieve pain
- Surgery is also appropriate if there is some expectation of improvement in function
- If, however, the pain level is mild to moderate and surgery is being undertaken with little expectation of functional improvement, careful weighing of risks and benefits is needed

---

Hip and knee replacement

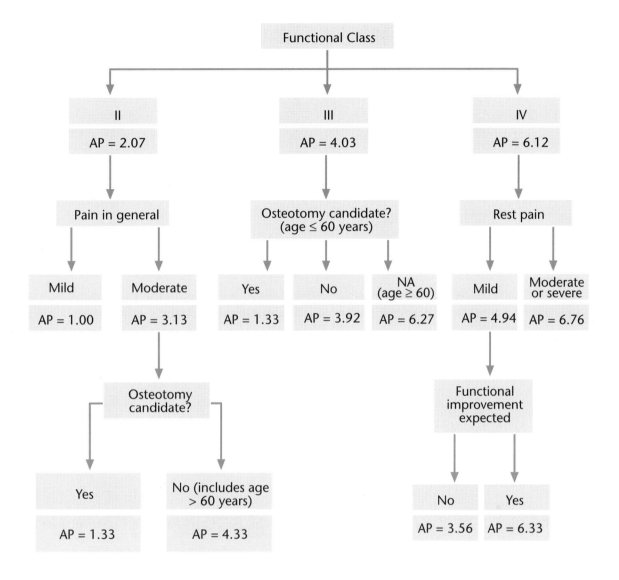

Appropriateness Scores (AP) range from 1 to 7

A score of 1 indicates that referral is inappropriate. The higher the score, the more the potential appropriateness for surgery. No cut off point was given, as appropriateness will vary according to resources in a given area. However, the implications from the text are that a score between 3–5 is still not conclusive, with other factors needing to be considered.

The original algorithm contained much extra statistical information. For simplicity, only the appropriateness score is retained in this version. It is actually the mean value of all the scores selected by the expert panel when asked to rate various scenarios in the different functional classes for appropriateness for GP referral.

Hip and knee replacement references

This guideline is based on:
Naylor CD and Williams JI (1996) Primary hip and knee replacement surgery: Ontario criteria for case selection and surgical priority. *Quality in Health Care*: **5**; 20–30.

Archroth P, Freeman MAR, Smillie IS *et al.* (1978) A knee function assessment chart. *J Bone Joint Surg*: **60B**; 308–10.

Bellamy N (1989) Pain assessment in osteoarthritis: experience with the WOMAC osteoarthritis index. *Sem Arthr Rheum*: **18**; 14–17.

Dorey F, Grigoris P and Amstutz H (1994) Making do without randomised trials. *J Bone Joint Surg*: **76B**; 1–3.

Kantz ME, Harris WJ, Levitsky K *et al.* (1992) Methods for assessing condition-specific and generic functional status outcomes after total knee replacement. *Med Care*: **30**; MS240–52.

Laupacis A, Bourne R, Rorabeck C *et al.* (1993) The effect of elective total hip replacement on health-related quality of life. *J Bone Joint Surg*: **75A**; 1619–26.

Liang MH and Jette AM (1981) Measuring functional ability in chronic arthritis. *Arthr Rheum*: **24**; 80–6.

Naylor CD (1995) Grey zones of clinical practice: some limits to evidence-based medicine. *Lancet*: **345**; 840–2.

Rajaratnam G, Black NA and Dalziel M (1990) Total hip replacements in the National Health Service: is need being met? *J Public Health Med*: **12**; 56–9.

Ranawat CS, Padgett DE and Ohashi Y (1989) Total knee arthroplasty for patients younger than 55 years. *Clin Orthop*: **248**; 27–33.

Surin VV and Sundholm K (1983) Survival of patients and prostheses after total hip arthroplasty. *Clin Orthop*: **177**; 148–53.

Williams MH, Newton JN, Frankel SJ *et al.* (1994) Prevalence of total hip replacement: how much demand has been met? *J Epidemol Comm Health*: **48**; 188–91.

Wright JG, Coyte PC, Hawker G *et al.* (1995) Variation in orthopedic surgeons' perceptions of the indications for and outcomes of knee replacement. *Can Med Assoc J*: **152**; 687–97.

Hyperlipidaemia

Hyperlipidaemia

Screening and diagnosis

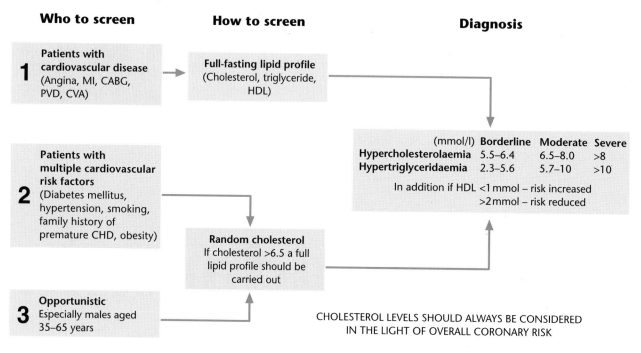

Who to screen

1 Patients with cardiovascular disease (Angina, MI, CABG, PVD, CVA)

2 Patients with multiple cardiovascular risk factors (Diabetes mellitus, hypertension, smoking, family history of premature CHD, obesity)

3 Opportunistic Especially males aged 35–65 years

How to screen

Full-fasting lipid profile (Cholesterol, triglyceride, HDL)

Random cholesterol If cholesterol >6.5 a full lipid profile should be carried out

Diagnosis

(mmol/l)	Borderline	Moderate	Severe
Hypercholesterolaemia	5.5–6.4	6.5–8.0	>8
Hypertriglyceridaemia	2.3–5.6	5.7–10	>10

In addition if HDL <1 mmol – risk increased
>2 mmol – risk reduced

CHOLESTEROL LEVELS SHOULD ALWAYS BE CONSIDERED IN THE LIGHT OF OVERALL CORONARY RISK

Management

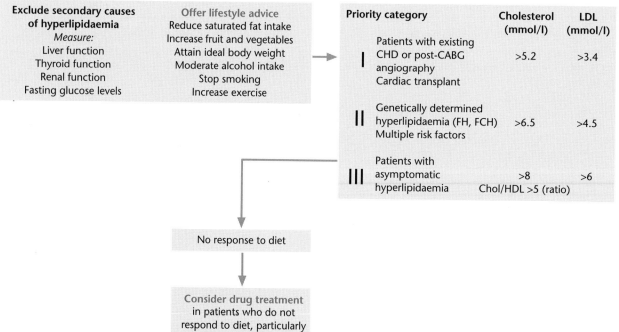

Exclude secondary causes of hyperlipidaemia
Measure:
Liver function
Thyroid function
Renal function
Fasting glucose levels

Offer lifestyle advice
Reduce saturated fat intake
Increase fruit and vegetables
Attain ideal body weight
Moderate alcohol intake
Stop smoking
Increase exercise

No response to diet

Consider drug treatment in patients who do not respond to diet, particularly in priority groups I and II

Intervention levels

Priority category	Cholesterol (mmol/l)	LDL (mmol/l)
I Patients with existing CHD or post-CABG angiography Cardiac transplant	>5.2	>3.4
II Genetically determined hyperlipidaemia (FH, FCH) Multiple risk factors	>6.5	>4.5
III Patients with asymptomatic hyperlipidaemia	>8 Chol/HDL >5 (ratio)	>6

Recommended therapeutic options

Indications	Drug	Contraindications
Hypercholesterolaemia (+/– raised triglyceride)	1 HMG CoA reductase inhibitor: simvastatin, pravastatin, fluvastatin	Liver disease, fertile females Extreme caution with cyclosporin
	2 Anion exchange resin: cholestyramine, colestipol	Hypertriglyceridaemia, peptic ulcer, haemorrhoids
	3 Fibrate: bezafibrate, ciprofibrate, fenofibrate, gemfibrozil	Renal failure, gallstones
Hypertriglyceridaemia (+/– raised cholesterol)	1 Fibrate	As above
	2 Nicotinic acid	Liver disease, gout, diabetes
Post-menopausal women Hypercholesterolaemia (+/– raised triglyceride)	1 HRT: Oral Transdermal Implant	Avoid oral route if triglyceride >2 mmol/l
	2 HMG CoA reductase inhibitor, Resin, Fibrate	

Treatment goals
Aim in patients with CHD is to reduce total cholesterol to <5.2 mmol/l
LDL – cholesterol to <3.4 mmol/l and reduce total cholesterol/HDL ratio to <5

Hospital referral
Patients with multiple pathology or unresponsive hyperlipidaemia can be referred to specialist clinics for initial investigation and management

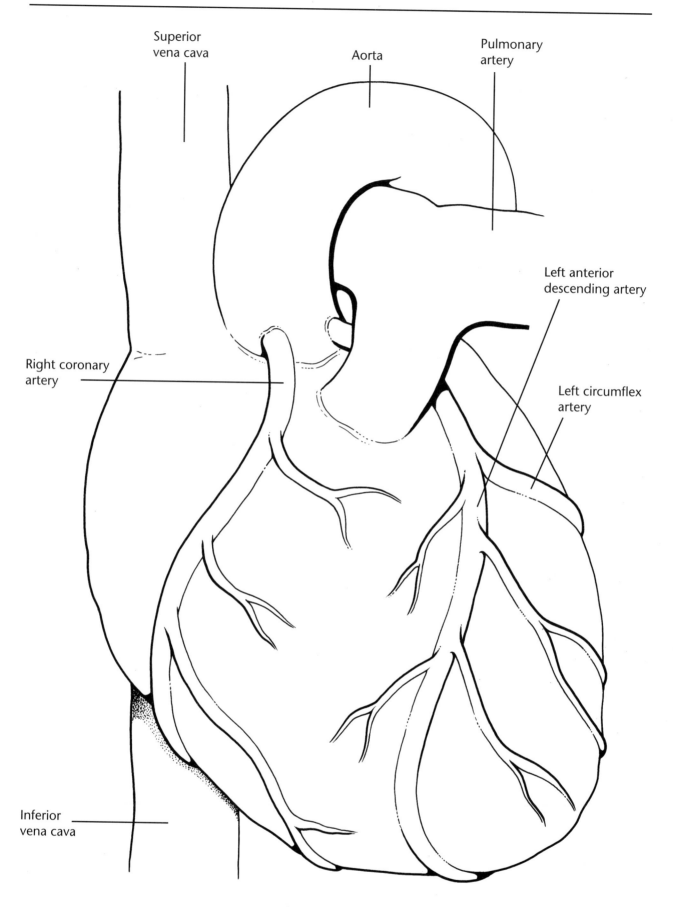

Superior
vena cava

Aorta

Pulmonary
artery

Left anterior
descending artery

Right coronary
artery

Left circumflex
artery

Inferior
vena cava

Figure 16.1 Main coronary arteries.

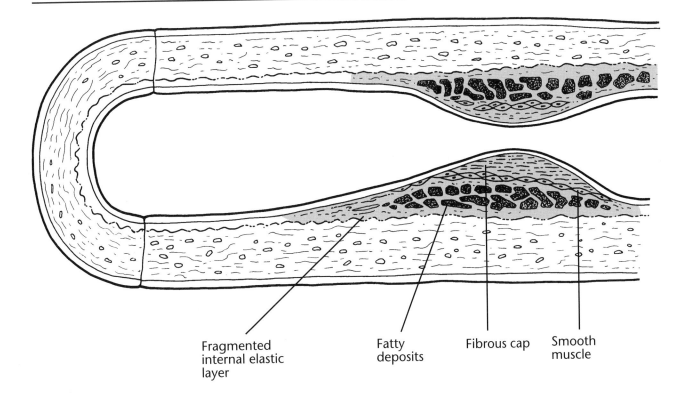

Fragmented
internal elastic
layer

Fatty
deposits

Fibrous cap

Smooth
muscle

Figure 16.2 Atheromatous plaque.

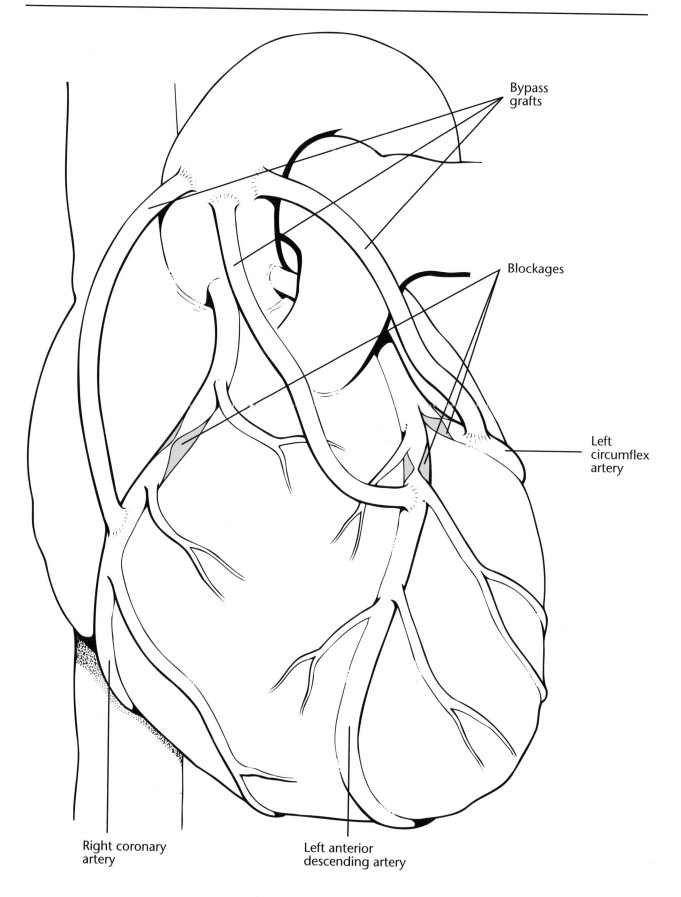

Figure 16.3 A 'triple bypass'.

Hyperlipidaemia references

This guideline is based on:
A simplified version of the British Hyperlipidaemia Association Guidelines. Betteridge *et al.* (1993) Management of hyperlipidaemia: guidelines of the British Hyperlipidaemia Association. *Postgrad Med J*: **69**; 359–69.

Davey Smith G, Song F and Sheldon TA (1993) Cholesterol lowering and the importance of considering initial level of risk. *BMJ*: **306**; 1367–73.

Harvard Atherosclerosis Reversibility Project (HARP) (1994) Effect on coronary atherosclerosis of decrease in plasma cholesterol in normocholesterolaemic patients. *Lancet*: **344**; 1182–6.

MAAS Investigators (1994) Effect of simvastatin on coronary atheroma: a multicentre antiatheroma study. *Lancet*: **344**; 633–8.

Oliver MF (1991) Might treatment of hypercholesterolaemia increase non-cardiac mortality? *Lancet*: **337**; 1529–31.

Oliver M, Poole-Wilson P, Shepherd J *et al.* (1995) Lower patients' cholesterol now. *BMJ*: **310**; 1280–1.

Pritchard BNC, Smith CCT, Ling KLE *et al.* (1995) Fish oils and cardiovascular risk. *BMJ*: **310**; 819–20.

Pyorala K, De Backer G, Poole-Wilson P *et al.* (1994) Prevention of coronary heart disease in clinical practice. Recommendations of the task force of the European Society of Cardiology, European Atherosclerosis Society and European Society of Hypertension. *Eur Heart J*: **15**; 1300–31.

Ramsey LE, Haq IU, Jackson PR and Yeo WW (1996) The Sheffield table for primary prevention of coronary heart disease: corrected. *Lancet*: **348**; 1251–2.

Rossouw JE, Lewis B and Rifkind BM (1990) The value of lowering cholesterol after myocardial infarction. *N Engl J Med*: **323**; 1112–9.

Sacks FM, Pfeffer MA, Moye LA *et al.* (1996) The effect of pravastatin on coronary events after myocardial infarction in patients with average cholesterol levels. Cholesterol and Recurrent Events (CARE) Trial. *New Engl J Med*: **335**; 1001–9.

Scandinavian Simvastatin Survival Study Group (1994) Randomised trial of cholesterol lowering in 4444 patients with coronary heart disease: the Scandinavian simvastatin survival study (4S). *Lancet*: **344**; 1383–9.

Shepherd J, Cobbe SM, Ford I (1995) Prevention of coronary heart disease with pravastatin in men with hypercholesterolaemia. West of Scotland Coronary Prevention Study Group (WOSCOPS). *New Engl J Med*: **333**; 1301–7.

Waters D, Higginson L, Gladstone P *et al.* (1994) Effects of monotherapy with an HMGCoA reductase inhibitor on the progression of coronary atherosclerosis as assessed by serial quantitative arteriography: the Canadian coronary atherosclerosis intervention trial. *Circulation*: **89**; 959–68.

Hypertension

Essential hypertension

Diastolic blood pressure

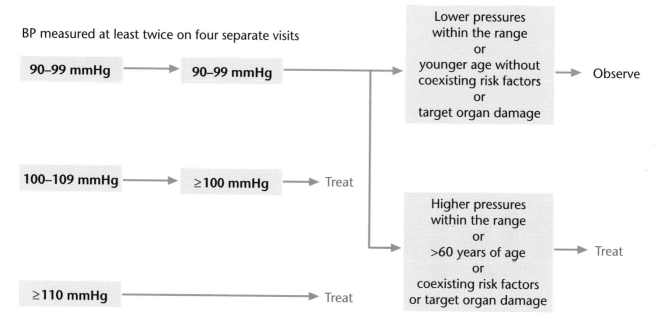

BP measured at least twice on four separate visits

90–99 mmHg → 90–99 mmHg

100–109 mmHg → ≥100 mmHg → Treat

≥110 mmHg → Treat

Lower pressures within the range
or
younger age without coexisting risk factors
or
target organ damage → Observe

Higher pressures within the range
or
>60 years of age
or
coexisting risk factors or target organ damage → Treat

Systolic blood pressure

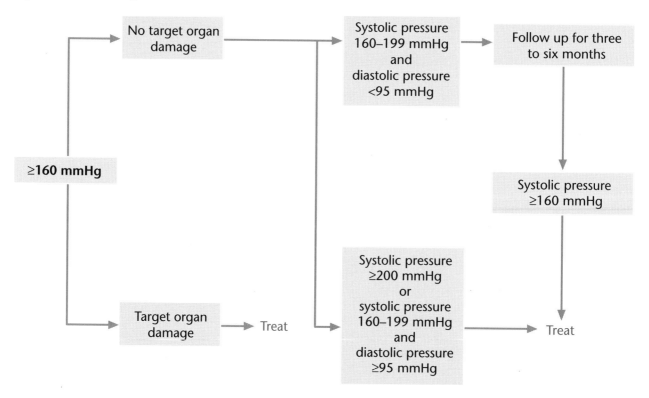

≥160 mmHg

No target organ damage → Systolic pressure 160–199 mmHg and diastolic pressure <95 mmHg → Follow up for three to six months

Systolic pressure ≥160 mmHg

Target organ damage → Treat

Systolic pressure ≥200 mmHg
or
systolic pressure 160–199 mmHg and diastolic pressure ≥95 mmHg → Treat

Essential hypertension
Choice of drugs

Co-existing disease	Diuretic	ß-blocker	ACE inhibitor	Calcium channel blocker	Alpha-blocker
Diabetes	Care needed	Care needed	Yes	Yes	Yes
Gout	No	Yes	Yes	Yes	Yes
Dyslipidaemia	Controversial	Controversial	Yes	Yes	Yes
Ischaemic heart disease	Yes	Yes	Yes	Yes	Yes
Heart failure	Yes	No	Yes	Care needed	Yes
Asthma	Yes	No	Yes	Yes	Yes
Collagen vascular disease	Yes	Care needed	Care needed	Yes	Yes
Renal artery stenosis	Yes	Yes	No	Yes	Yes

Essential hypertension

Treatment

Goals
Diastolic – reduce to <90 mmHg
Systolic – probably prudent to reduce to <160 mmHg
Non-pharmacological measures recommended to all hypertensives
and to all people with a strong family history of hypertension

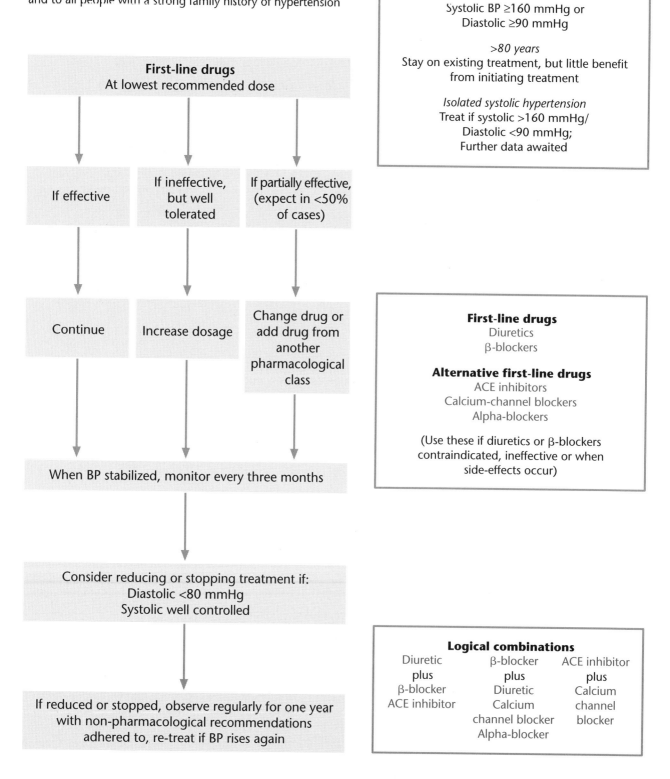

The elderly
60–80 years
Treat if
Systolic BP ≥160 mmHg or
Diastolic ≥90 mmHg

>80 years
Stay on existing treatment, but little benefit
from initiating treatment

Isolated systolic hypertension
Treat if systolic >160 mmHg/
Diastolic <90 mmHg;
Further data awaited

First-line drugs
At lowest recommended dose

If effective

If ineffective,
but well
tolerated

If partially effective,
(expect in <50%
of cases)

Continue

Increase dosage

Change drug or
add drug from
another
pharmacological
class

When BP stabilized, monitor every three months

Consider reducing or stopping treatment if:
Diastolic <80 mmHg
Systolic well controlled

If reduced or stopped, observe regularly for one year
with non-pharmacological recommendations
adhered to, re-treat if BP rises again

First-line drugs
Diuretics
β-blockers

Alternative first-line drugs
ACE inhibitors
Calcium-channel blockers
Alpha-blockers

(Use these if diuretics or β-blockers
contraindicated, ineffective or when
side-effects occur)

Logical combinations
Diuretic	β-blocker	ACE inhibitor
plus	plus	plus
β-blocker	Diuretic	Calcium
ACE inhibitor	Calcium	channel
	channel blocker	blocker
	Alpha-blocker	

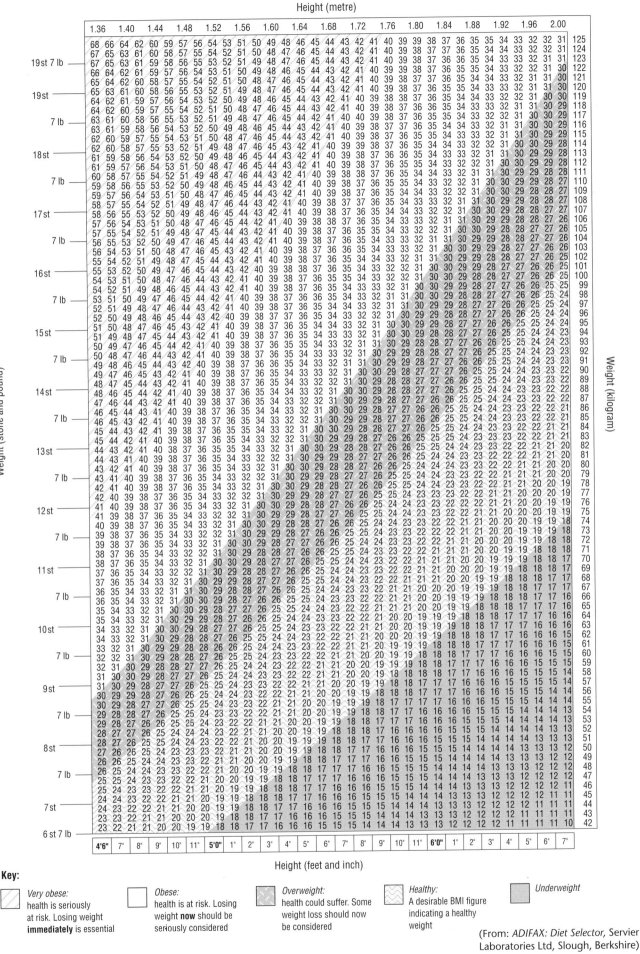

Figure 17.1 Body mass index ready reckoner.

Key:

Very obese: health is seriously at risk. Losing weight **immediately** is essential

Obese: health is at risk. Losing weight **now** should be seriously considered

Overweight: health could suffer. Some weight loss should now be considered

Healthy: A desirable BMI figure indicating a healthy weight

Underweight

(From: ADIFAX: Diet Selector, Servier Laboratories Ltd, Slough, Berkshire)

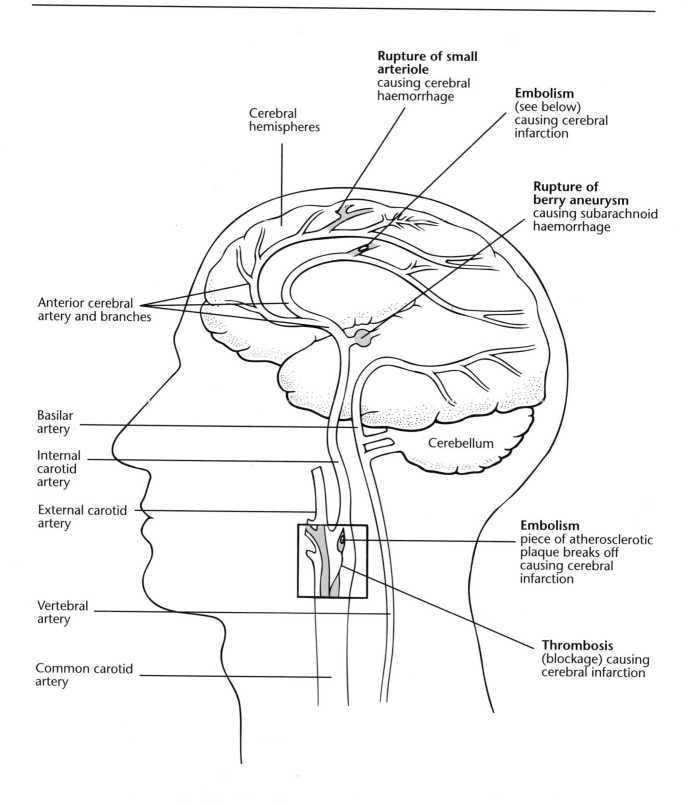

Figure 17.2 How hypertension can cause strokes.

Hypertension references

This guideline is based on:
A simplified version of the British Hypertension Society Guidelines in: Sever *et al.* (1993) Management guidelines in essential hypertension: report of the second working party of the British Hypertension Society. *BMJ*: **306**; 983–8.

Amery A, Birkenhäger W, Brixko P *et al.* (1985) Mortality and morbidity results from the European Working Party on High Blood Pressure in the Elderly trial. *Lancet*: **i**; 1349–54.

Dahlöf B, Hansson L, Lindholm L *et al.* (1993) STOP-Hypertension 2. Swedish trial in old patients with hypertension. *Blood Pressure*: **2(2)**; 136–41.

Dahlöf B, Lindholm L, Hansson L *et al.* (1991) Morbidity and mortality in the Swedish Trial in Old Patients with Hypertension. (STOP-Hypertension). *Lancet*: **338**; 1281–5.

Fahey TP and Peters TJ (1996) What constitutes controlled hypertension? Patient based comparison of hypertension guidelines. *BMJ*: **313**; 93–6.

Furberg CD (1995) Nifedipine: dose-related increase in mortality in patients with coronary heart disease. *Circulation*: **92**; 1326–31.

Haynes RB, Sackett DL, Taylor DW *et al.* (1978) Increased absenteeism from work after detection and labelling of hypertensive patients. *N Engl J Med*: **299**; 741–4.

Medical Research Council Working Party (1985) MRC trial of treatment of mild hypertension: principal results. *BMJ*: **291**; 97–104.

MRC Working Party (1992) Medical Research Council trial on treatment of hypertension in older adults: principal results. *BMJ*: **304**; 405–12.

SHEP Cooperative Research Group (1991) Prevention of stroke by antihypertensive drug treatment in older persons with isolated systolic hypertension. *JAMA*: **265**; 3255–64.

Swales JD (1994) Pharmacological treatment of hypertension. *Lancet*: **334**; 380–5.

The HOT Study Group (1992) The Hypertension Optimal Treatment Study (The HOT-Study). *Blood Pressure*: **2**; 62–8.

The SOLVD Investigators (1992) Effect of enalapril on mortality and the development of heart failure in asymptomatic patients with reduced left ventricular ejection fraction. *N Engl J Med*: **327**; 685–91.

Infertility

Infertility

Female

History

Female menstrual history including:
Cycle length (<21 days, 22–42 days, >42 days)
Irregularity of menstrual cycle –
amenorrhoea
Oligomenorrhoea (cycle length >42 days)
Dysmenorrhoea
Sexual – dyspareunia, coital history
IMB or PCB
Medical history, including on-going systemic
illness
Gynaecological history, including ectopic
pregnancy, suspected or proven PID and STD
and gynaecological operations
Other abdominal operations

Examination

Hirsutism
Galactorrhoea
Other signs of endocrine disorder
Height and weight
Pelvic and abdominal examination

Pre-referral investigation

All women
Rubella status if not known
Haemoglobin if menorrhagia, dietary restriction
or otherwise clinically indicated
Thalassaemia and sickle cell if from outside
Northern Europe. (If positive, test partner whatever
his origins)

Amenorrhoeic

LH/FSH at any time
(Progesterone not required)
TSH
Prolactin

**Cycle <21 days or between
21–42 days**
LH/FSH between days one to
five of cycle
Progesterone seven days
before menstruation or (if
using ovulation predictor kit)
eight days after LH surge

Cycle length >42 days

LH/FSH between days one to
five of cycle
TSH
Prolactin
(Progesterone not required)

Male

History

Any pregnancies fathered?
Previous illness (particularly pyrexial illness within
last six months)
Orchitis, epididymitis, torsion, maldescent,
varicocoele
Treatment of above illness, at what age and
whether surgical
Sexual – ejaculation, erection, coital frequency
STD
Smoking
Alcohol use

Examination

Testicular site and volume
Varicocoele
Epididymal thickening
Scrotal swelling
Other signs of urogenital abnormality

Pre-referral investigation

Semen analysis

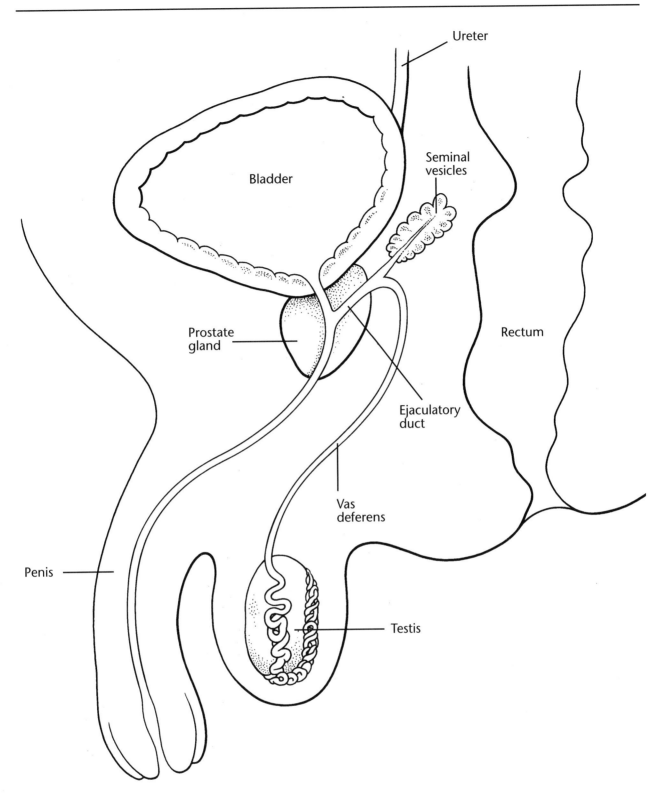

Figure 18.1   Normal male reproductive system.

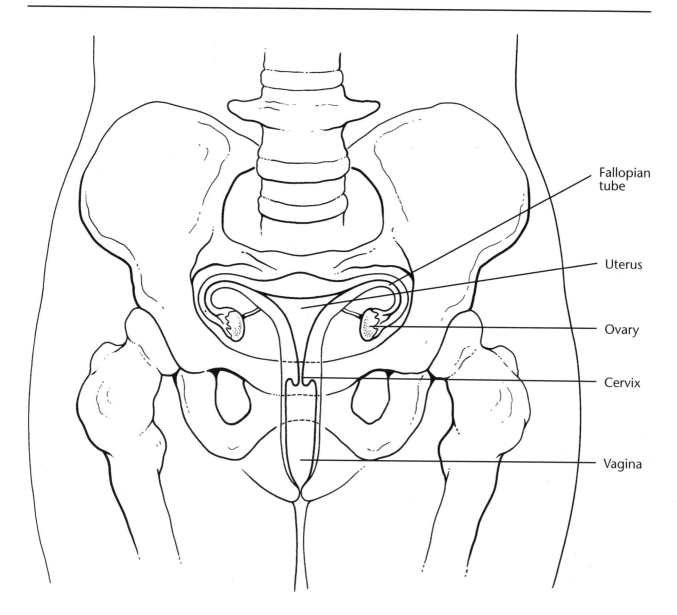

Fallopian tube

Uterus

Ovary

Cervix

Vagina

Figure 18.2   Female reproductive organs in relation to the pelvic bones.

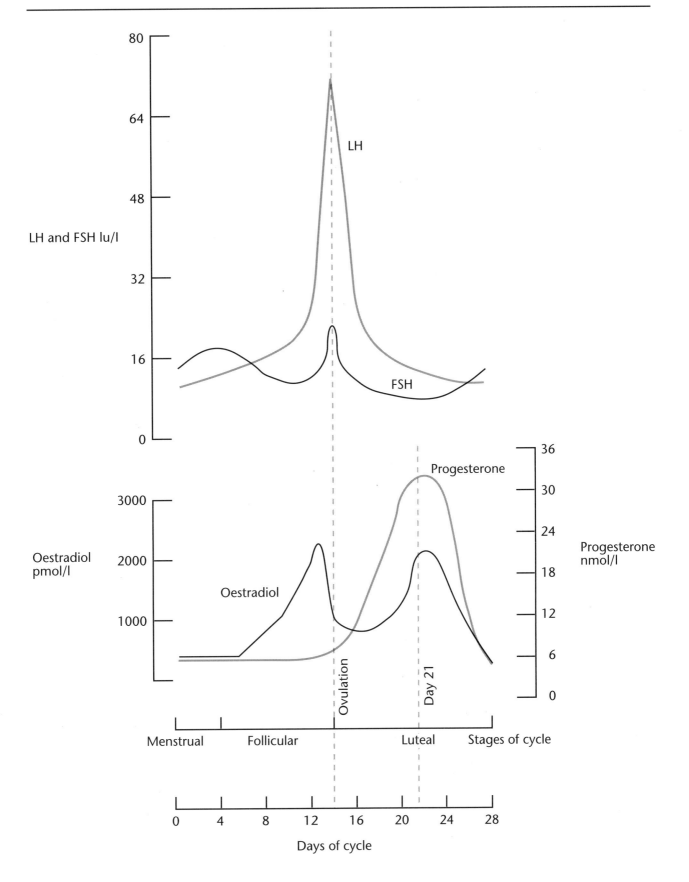

Figure 18.3 Hormonal changes during normal menstrual cycle.

Infertility references

This guideline was developed using:
Royal College of Obstetricians and Gynaecologists (1992) *Infertility Guidelines for Practice*. RCOG Press, London.

American Fertility Society (1990) New guidelines for the use of semen for donor insemination 1990. *Fertil Steril*: **53**(Suppl. 1); 1S–13S.

Asch RH, Balmaceda JP, Ellsworth LR *et al.* (1985) Gamete Intra-Fallopian Transfer (GIFT): A new treatment for infertility. *Int J Fertil*: **30**; 41–5.

Edwards RG (ed.) (1990) Assisted Human Conception. Special review in *Med Bull*: **46**; 567–864. Published by Churchill Livingstone for the British Council.

Gomaa A, Shalaby M, Osman M *et al.* (1996) Topical treatment of erectile dysfunction: randomised double blind placebo controlled trial of cream containing aminophylline, isosorbide dinitrate and co-dergocrine mesylate. *BMJ*: **312**; 1512–14.

Jequier A (1986) Infertility in the male. *Current Reviews in Obstetrics and Gynaecology*. Churchill Livingstone, Edinburgh.

Mahmood TA and Templeton A (1990) The impact of treatment on the natural history of endometriosis. *Hum Repro*: **5**; 965–70.

Rai R, Cohen H, Dare M *et al.* (1997) Randomised controlled trial of aspirin and aspirin plus heparin in pregnant women with recurrent miscarriage associated with phospholipid antibodies (or antiphospholipid antibodies) *BMJ*: **313**; 239–314.

Royal College of Obstetricians and Gynaecologists (1992) *Important Information for Semen Donors*: *Donor Insemination*: *Patient Information Booklet*. Royal College of Obstetricians and Gynaecologists, London.

Snowden R and E (1984) *The Gift of a Child*. Allen and Unwin, London.

Thomas EJ (1991) Endometriosis and infertility. In *Modern Approaches to Endometriosis*. (eds EJ Thomas and J Rock) Kluwer Academic Publishers, Lancaster, pp. 113–28.

Thomas EJ and Prentice A (1992) The aetiology and pathogenesis of endometriosis, *Repro Med Rev*: **1**; 21–36.

Winston RML and Margara RA (1991) Microsurgical salpingostomy is not an obsolete procedure. *Br J Obstet Gynaecol*: **98**; 637–42.

Inflammatory Bowel Disease

Inflammatory bowel disease

When to suspect a diagnosis of inflammatory bowel disease

Ulcerative colitis
Rectal bleeding with mucus, urgency and bowel frequency (stools can be solid)
Persistent watery diarrhoea
Rectal bleeding starting after stopping smoking
Commonest age of presentation: young adults. If >50, symptoms more likely to be due to colonic cancer, but could still be due to UC

Crohn's disease
Diarrhoea, abdominal pain and weight loss or growth failure
Nocturnal diarrhoea
Systemic disturbance (fever; malaise)
Above symptoms with peri-anal disease (fissures, fistulae, abscesses, fleshy tags)

Suspect IBD if
Patient presents with diarrhoea or abdominal pain and one or more of the following:
Mouth ulcers, iritis, episcleritis, clubbing, erythema nodosum, pyoderma, arthropathy
Family history of IBD or ankylosing spondylitis
Abnormal screening investigations suggesting possible IBD (see below)

Examination and investigations

Examination should include:
Abdominal palpation
Anal inspection
Digital rectal examination
Endoscopy if facilities available

The following results may indicate IBD:
Platelet count – ↑
FBC – Hb↓, WBC↑
ESR – ↑
Albumin – ↓

CRP – ↑
Plasma viscosity – ↑
Stool cultures – neg.

Bilirubin, alkaline phosphatase, alanine transaminase – ↑ if hepatic involvement
No Ba enema unless digital rectal and at least sigmoidoscopy performed

Hospital referral

When to refer the suspected new patient
Urgent referral should be made to a hospital consultant when the diagnosis is suspected
If abdominal pain and particularly abdominal tenderness, severe diarrhoea with bleeding, or fever, refer immediately for possible admission

Long-term follow up

Follow-up of ulcerative colitis

Hospital doctor
Extensive or total UC even if quiescent (cancer risk). All should be reviewed after seven to ten years and seen annually for supervision and colonoscopy thereafter
Unstable disease patients with disease that relapses frequently and is steroid dependent
Patients on immunosuppressives – but GP may wish to undertake routine FBC monitoring

General practitioner
Proctitis or distal colitis with infrequent relapses
Quiescent colitis to splenic flexure, with infrequent relapses

Re-referral of patients with ulcerative colitis
Proctitis or distal ulcerative colitis, not settling with oral/rectal 5-ASA and/or rectal steroid foam or liquid enema
More extensive colitis getting worse (immediate, for possible admission), featuring: watery/bloody diarrhoea >8 per day, fever, tachycardia, pain, weight loss, thirst, anaemia, systemic accompaniments – patient looks ill enough to need systemic steroids
Poor response to systemic steroids
Recurrent need for systemic steroids
Suspicion of cancer
OR
Any other circumstances giving cause for concern

Follow-up of Crohn's disease

Hospital doctor
Complex extensive active disease – particularly those with nutritional problems, growth failure, systemic complications, peri-anal sepsis
Steroid dependent
Patients on immunosuppressives e.g. methotrexate, cyclosporin, azathioprine
Patients on special diets
Patients with ileal resections for annual B_{12} level check (or im B_{12} or GP if effective follow up)

General practitioner
Patients with previous diagnosis, but quiescent or low-grade symptoms

Re-referral of patients with Crohn's disease
Poor response to systemic steroids
Recurrent need for systemic steroids
Symptoms suggesting obstruction (vomiting, distension, colic)
Suspicion of cancer
OR
Any other circumstances giving cause for concern

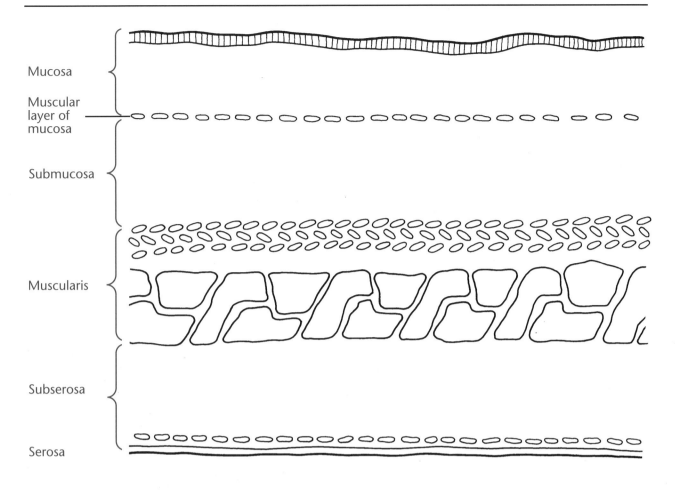

Mucosa

Muscular layer of mucosa

Submucosa

Muscularis

Subserosa

Serosa

Figure 19.1 Basic structure of wall of large bowel.

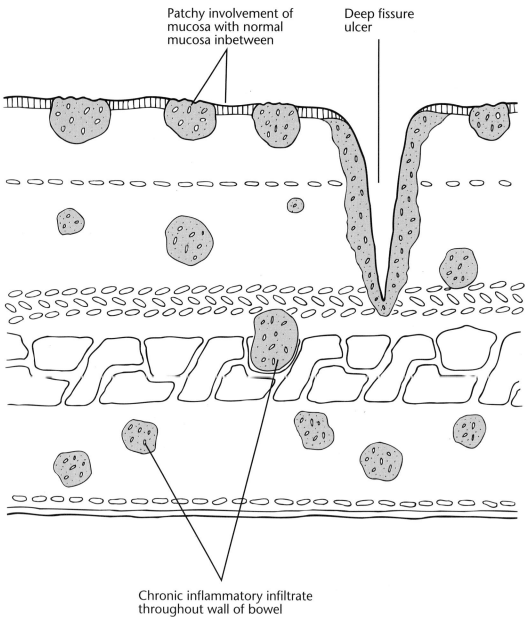

Patchy involvement of mucosa with normal mucosa inbetween

Deep fissure ulcer

Chronic inflammatory infiltrate throughout wall of bowel

Figure 19.2 Crohn's disease.

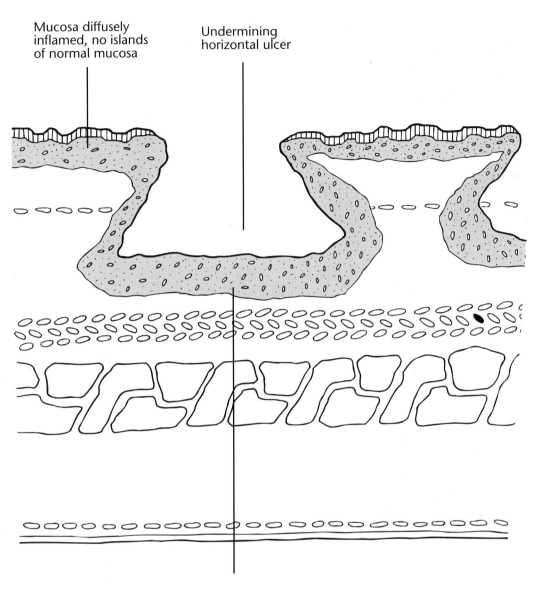

Mucosa diffusely inflamed, no islands of normal mucosa

Undermining horizontal ulcer

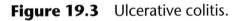

Generally ulcers no deeper than submucosa, with occasional deep ulcer involving muscle layer

Figure 19.3 Ulcerative colitis.

Inflammatory bowel disease references

This guideline is based on:
British Society of Gastroenterology (1996) *Guidelines in Gastroenterology: Inflammatory Bowel Disease Management Guidelines.* BSG, London. See Dyspepsia reference for details.

Binder V, Hendriksen C and Kreiner S (1985) Prognosis in Crohn's disease – based on results from a regional patient group from the country of Copenhagen. *Gut*: **26**; 146–50.

Cotton M, Rosselli, Orlando A *et al.* (1994) Smoking habits and recurrence of Crohn's disease. *Gastroenterol*: **106**; 643–8.

Ekbom A, Helmick CG, Zack M *et al.* (1992) Survival and causes of death in patients with inflammatory bowel disease: a population-based study. *Gastroenterol*: **103**; 954–60.

Griffiths AM, Ohlsson A, Sherman PM *et al.* (1995) Meta-analysis of enteral nutrition as a primary treatment of active Crohn's disease. *Gastroenterol*: **108**; 1056–67.

Hendriksen C, Kreiner S and Binder V (1985) Long term prognosis in ulcerative colitis – based on results from a regional patient group from the country of Copenhagen. *Gut*: **26**; 158–63.

Jewell DP (1989) Corticosteroids for the management of ulcerative colitis and Crohn's disease. *Gastroenterol Clin North Am*: **18**(1); 21–33.

Langholz E, Munkholm P, Davidsen M *et al.* (1992) Colorectal cancer risk and mortality in patients with ulcerative colitis. *Gastroenterol*: **103**; 1444–51.

Langholz E, Munkholm P, Davidsen M *et al.* (1994) Course of ulcerative colitis: analysis of changes in disease activity over years. *Gastroenterol*: **107**; 3–11.

Marshall JK and Irvine EJ (1995) Rectal aminosalicylate therapy for distal ulcerative colitis: a meta-analysis. *Alimen Pharmacol and Therapeut*: **9**(3); 293–300.

Munkholm P, Langholz E, Davidsen M *et al.* (1993) Intestinal cancer risk and mortality in patients with Crohn's disease. *Gastroenterol*: **105**; 1716–23.

Steinhart AH, Hemphill D and Greenberg GR (1994) Sulphasalazine and mesalazine for the maintenance therapy of Crohn's disease: a meta-analysis. *Amer J Gastroenterol*: **89**; 2116–24.

Sutherland LR, May GR and Shaffer EA (1993) Sulphasalazine revisited: a meta-analysis of 5-aminosalicylic acid in the treatment of ulcerative colitis. *Ann Intern Med*: **118**; 540–9.

20

Migraine

Migraine – initial strategy

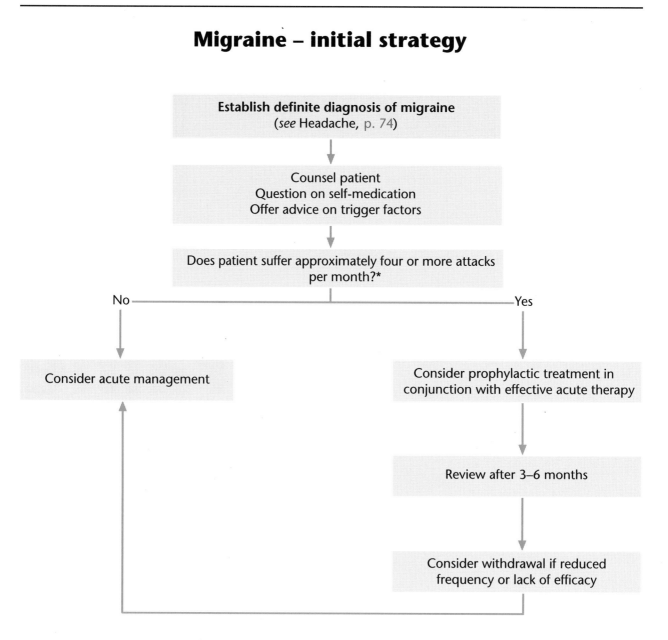

Establish definite diagnosis of migraine
(*see* Headache, p. 74)

Counsel patient
Question on self-medication
Offer advice on trigger factors

Does patient suffer approximately four or more attacks
per month?*

No — Yes

Consider acute management

Consider prophylactic treatment in
conjunction with effective acute therapy

Review after 3–6 months

Consider withdrawal if reduced
frequency or lack of efficacy

*Patients with less frequent but prolonged disabling attacks may warrant prophylaxis if their migraines are
unresponsive to sumatriptan

Migraine – overall strategy

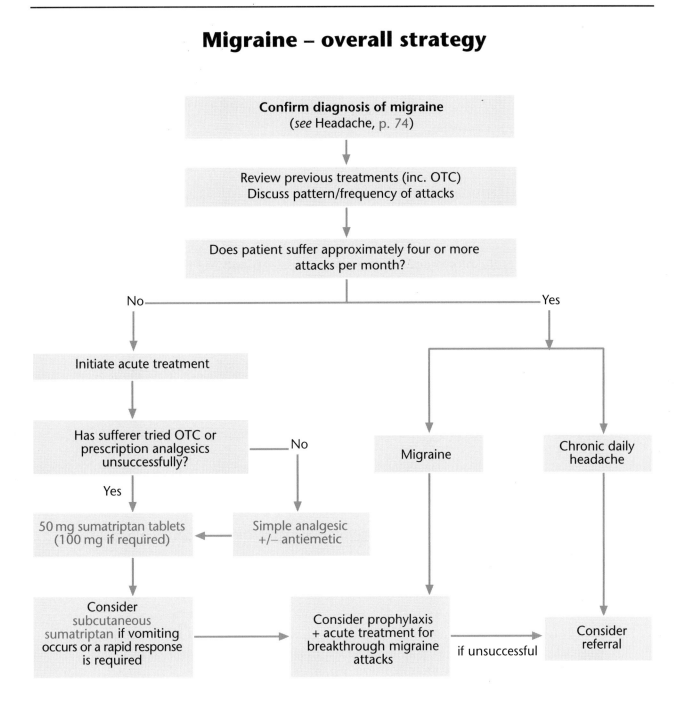

Migraine references

This guideline is based on:
MIPCA (1997) *A Strategy for the Modern Management of Migraine*. Published by Synergy Medical Education, 1 The Green, Richmond, Surrey. Reproduced with permission.

Anthony M, Hinterberger H and Lance JW (1969) The possible relationship of serotonin to the migraine syndrome. *Res Clin Stud Headache*: **2**; 29–59.

Blau JN (1982) Resolution of migraine attacks: sleep and the recovery phase. *J Neurol Neurosurg Psychiat*: **45**; 223–6.

Blau JN and Drummond MF (1991) *Migraine*. Office of Health Economics, London.

Curran DA, Hinterberger H and Lance JW (1965) Total plasma serotonin, 5-hydroxy-indoleacetic acid and p-hydroxy-m-methoxymandelic acid excretion in normal and migrainous subjects. *Brain*: **88**; 997 1010.

Goadsby PJ and Oleson J (1996) Diagnosis and management of migraine. *BMJ*: **312**; 1279–83.

Graham JR and Wolff HG (1938) Mechanism of migraine headache and action of ergotamine tartrate. *Arch Neurol Psychiat*: **39**; 737–63.

Humphrey PPA (1991) 5-Hydroxytryptamine and the pathophysiology of migraine. *J Neurol*: **238**; S38–S44.

Lipton RB and Stewart WF (1994) The epidemiology of migraine. *Eur Neurol*: **34** (Suppl. 2); 6–11.

Moskowitz MA (1987) Sensory connections to cephalic blood vessels and their possible importance to vascular headaches. In *Advances in Headache Research*. (ed. F Clifford-Rose) John Libbey, London, pp. 81–6.

Sicuteri F (1967) Vasoneuractive substances and their implication in vascular pain. *Res Clin Stud Headache*: **1**; 6–45.

Sicuteri F, Testi A and Anselmi B (1961) Biochemical investigations in headache: increase in hydroxyindoleacetic acid excretion during migraine attacks. *Int Arch Allergy Appl Immunol*: **19**; 55–8.

van Zwieten PA, Blauw G and van Brummelen P (1990) Pathophysiological and pharmacotherapeutic aspects of serotonin and serotonergic drugs. *Clin Physiol Biochem*: **8** (Suppl. 3); 1–18.

21

Oesophageal Reflux and Oesophagitis

Oesophageal reflux

Management prior to hospital investigation

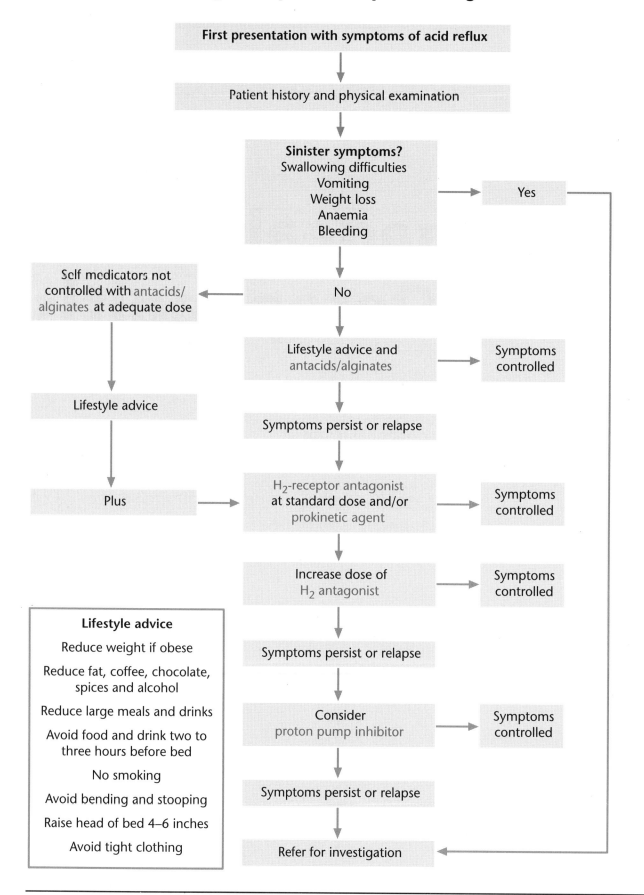

First presentation with symptoms of acid reflux

Patient history and physical examination

Sinister symptoms?
Swallowing difficulties
Vomiting
Weight loss
Anaemia
Bleeding

Yes

Self medicators not controlled with antacids/ alginates at adequate dose

No

Lifestyle advice and antacids/alginates

Symptoms controlled

Lifestyle advice

Symptoms persist or relapse

Plus

H_2-receptor antagonist at standard dose and/or prokinetic agent

Symptoms controlled

Increase dose of H_2 antagonist

Symptoms controlled

Lifestyle advice

Reduce weight if obese

Reduce fat, coffee, chocolate, spices and alcohol

Reduce large meals and drinks

Avoid food and drink two to three hours before bed

No smoking

Avoid bending and stooping

Raise head of bed 4–6 inches

Avoid tight clothing

Symptoms persist or relapse

Consider
proton pump inhibitor

Symptoms controlled

Symptoms persist or relapse

Refer for investigation

Oesophagitis

Management after endoscopy

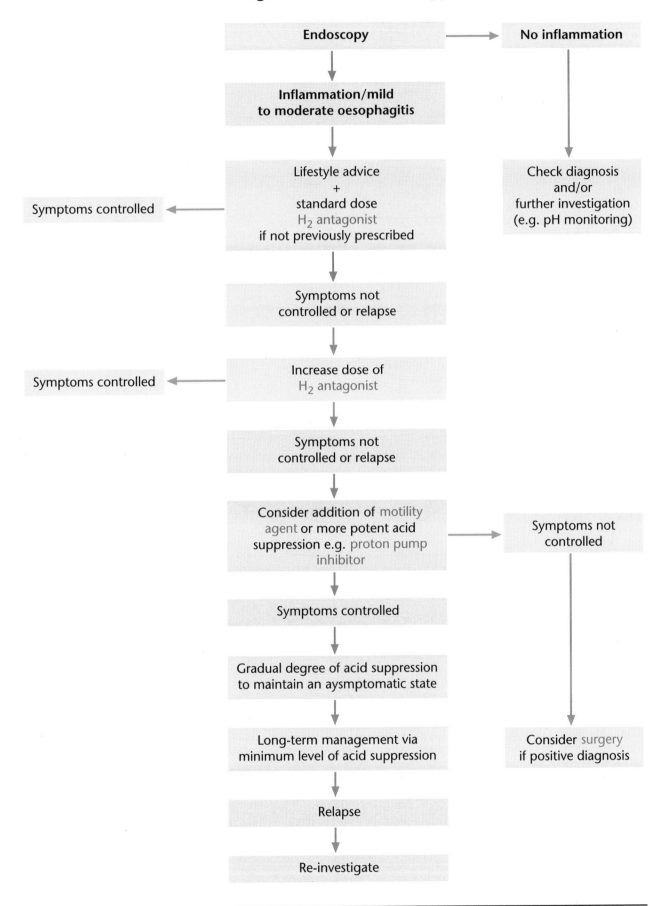

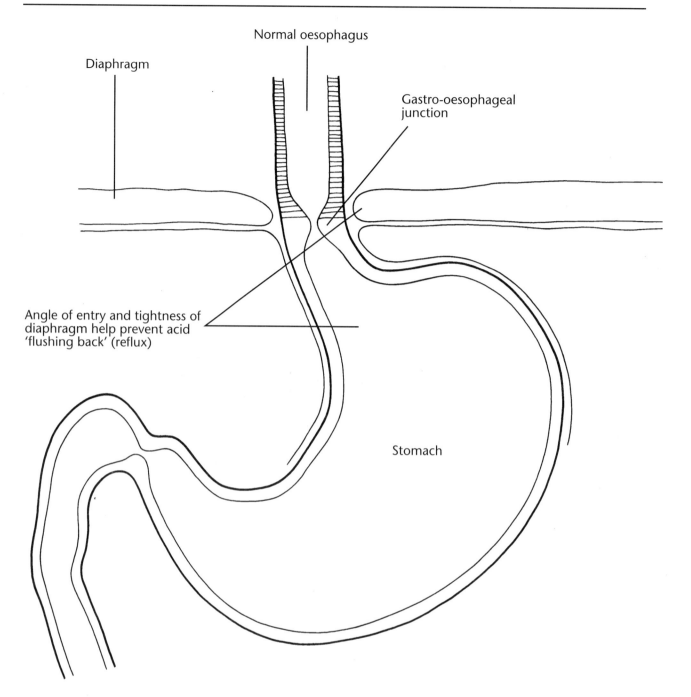

Diaphragm

Normal oesophagus

Gastro-oesophageal junction

Angle of entry and tightness of diaphragm help prevent acid 'flushing back' (reflux)

Stomach

Figure 21.1 Normal stomach and oesophagus.

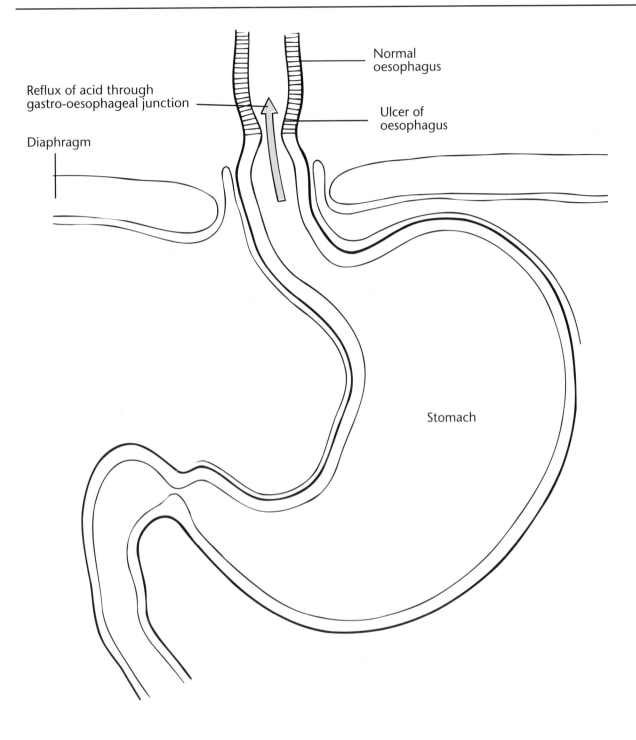

Figure 21.2 Sliding hiatus hernia showing reflux.

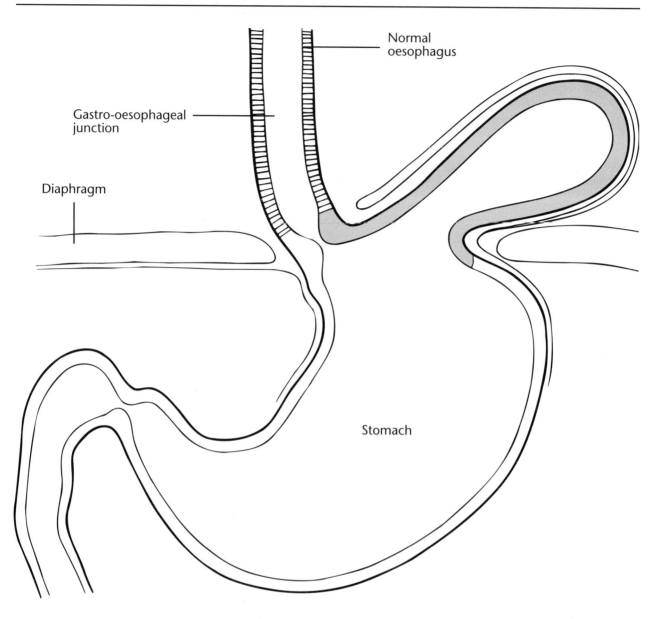

Normal oesophagus

Gastro-oesophageal junction

Diaphragm

Stomach

Figure 21.3 Paraoesophageal hiatus hernia.

Oesophageal reflux and oesophagitis references

This guideline is based on:
Management Guidelines for Gastro-oesophageal Reflux Disease, from a round table discussion at the European Digestive Week, Amsterdam, October, 1991.

Axon AT, Bell GD, Quine MA *et al.* (1995) Guidelines on the appropriate indications for upper gastrointestinal endoscopy. Working Party of the Joint Committee of the Royal College of Physicians of London, Royal College of Surgeons of England, Royal College of Anaesthetists, Association of Surgeons, the British Society of Gastroenterology and the Thoracic Society of Great Britain. *BMJ*: **310**; 816–17.

British Society of Gastroenterology (1996) *Guidelines in Gastroenterology: 1: Dyspepsia Management Guidelines*. BSG, London.

Bytzer P, Moller Hansen J and Schaffalitzky de Muckadeil OB (1994) Empirical H$_2$-blocker therapy or prompt endoscopy in management of dyspepsia. *Lancet*: **343**; 811–6.

Colin-Jones DG (1988) Management of dyspepsia: report of a working party. *Lancet*: **(i)**; 576–9.

Gough AL, Long RG, Cooper BT *et al.* (1996) Lansoprazole versus ranitidine in the maintenance treatment of reflux oesophagitis. *Aliment Pharmacol Ther*: **10**; 529–39.

Goulston KJ, Dent OF, Mant A *et al.* (1991) Use of H$_2$ receptor antagonists in patients with dyspepsia and heartburn: a cost comparison. *Med J Aust*: **155**; 20–6.

Jones R (1988) What happens to patients with non-ulcer dyspepsia after endoscopy? *Practitioner*: **232**; 75–8.

Jones RH, Lydeard SE, Hobbs FSR *et al.* (1990) Dyspepsia in England and Scotland. *Gut*: **31**; 40–5.

Johnston BJ, Reed PI and DG Newell (1990) How to reduce the endoscopic workload. *Gut*: **3**; A613.

Nyren O, Lindberg G, Lindstrom E *et al.* (1992) Economic costs of functional dyspepsia. *Pharm Econ*: **1**; 312–24.

Quine MA, Bell GD, McCloy RF *et al.* (1994) Appropriate use of upper gastrointestinal endoscopy – a prospective audit. *Gut*: **35**; 1209–14.

Talley NJ, Colin-Jones D, Koch IK *et al.* (1991) Functional dyspepsia: a classification with guidelines for diagnosis and management. *Gastroenterol Int*: **4**; 145–60.

22

Osteoporosis

Osteoporosis

Clinical triggers
Early menopause: <45 years (either surgical or natural)
Premenopausal amenorrhoea
Low trauma fracture (Colles', vertebrae, hip)
Back pain
Loss of height
Kyphosis
Steroids

Yes

Clinical assessment
Other risk factors and secondary causes
Differential diagnosis (X-ray, biochemistry/haematology refer for specialist opinion) (see p. 131)
Contraindications to treatment
Identify targets for lifestyle advice

Refer for bone densitometry

Risk factors

Modifiable:	*Non-modifiable:*
Oestrogen deficiency syndromes	Age
Smoking	Nulliparity
Alcohol abuse	Race – Caucasian or Asian
Prolonged immobilization/ inactivity	Positive family history
Some drugs	Prior fragility fracture
Nutritional deficiencies	Short stature and small bones
Certain diseases (see p. 131)	
Low body-mass index	
Susceptibility to falls	

Lifestyle changes
Stop smoking
Reduce alcohol intake
Regular weight-bearing exercise
Improve levels of calcium and vitamin D in the diet
Test eyesight
Review long-acting psychotropic medication
Examine home for obstacles that may increase the chances of sustaining a fall

Management
Lifestyle advice (consideration and counselling with regard to other modifiable risk structures) will benefit all patients

Pharmacological intervention
HRT
Calcium and vitamin D
Biphosphonates if vertebral fracture
Analgesia/NSAIDS
Physiotherapy

Osteoporosis

Causes of secondary osteoporosis

Endocrine disease/metabolic causes:

Hypogonadism

Hyperadrenocorticism (e.g. Cushing's Syndrome, excessive steroid therapy)

Hyperparathyroidism

Thyrotoxicosis

Anorexia nervosa

Hyperprolactinaemia

Nutritional causes

Malabsorption syndromes/malnutrition

Chronic liver disease

Vitamin D deficiency

Alcoholism

Gastric surgery

Drugs

Corticosteroids

Chronic heparin administration

Other

Osteogenesis imperfecta

Rheumatoid arthritis

Myeloma and some cancers

Prolonged immobilization

Investigations to identify secondary causes of osteoporosis

Blood tests:	*Urine tests:*
FBC, ESR, U&E, LFTs	(if raised ESR)
Calcium, phosphate, alkaline phosphatase	Bence Jones protein
Immunoglobulins (if ESR elevated)	
TFTs	*24 hour urine for:*
Testosterone (in men)	Calcium
Plasma electrophoresis	Creatinine

Indications for bone densitometry referrals

(only if an investigation result is important in the management decision)

Early surgical or natural menopause (<45 years)

Premenopausal amenorrhoea (<six months)

Vertebral fracture low trauma (only refer if doubt about level of trauma involved or underlying pathology)

Colles' fracture, low trauma (fall from standing height or less)

Steroid use (e.g. >7.5 mg/day prednisolone)

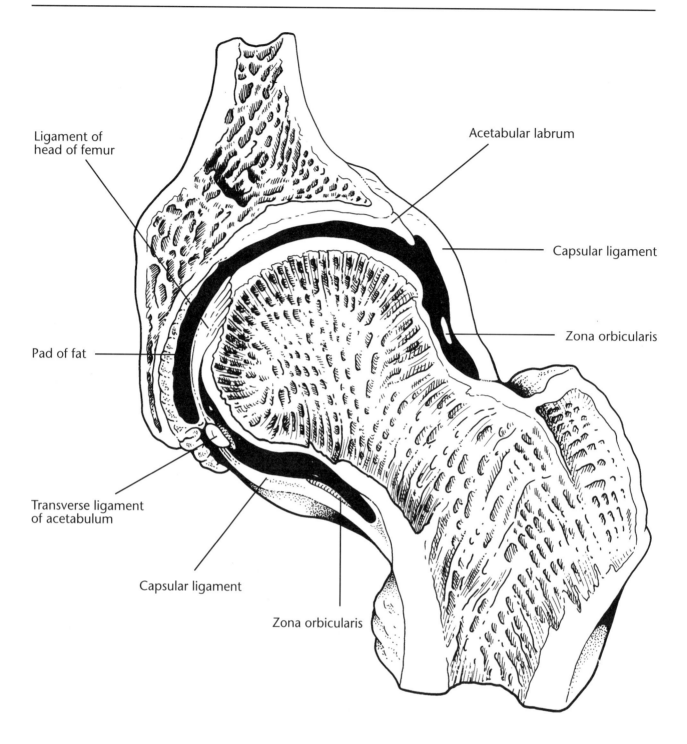

Ligament of
head of femur

Acetabular labrum

Capsular ligament

Pad of fat

Zona orbicularis

Transverse ligament
of acetabulum

Capsular ligament

Zona orbicularis

Figure 22.1   Section through the hip joint.

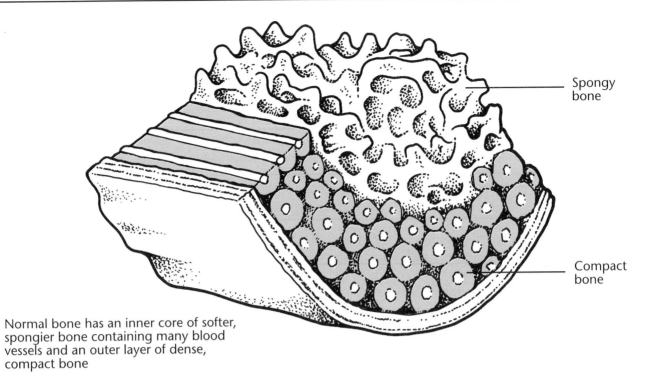

Normal bone has an inner core of softer, spongier bone containing many blood vessels and an outer layer of dense, compact bone

Spongy bone

Compact bone

Figure 22.2   Normal bone.

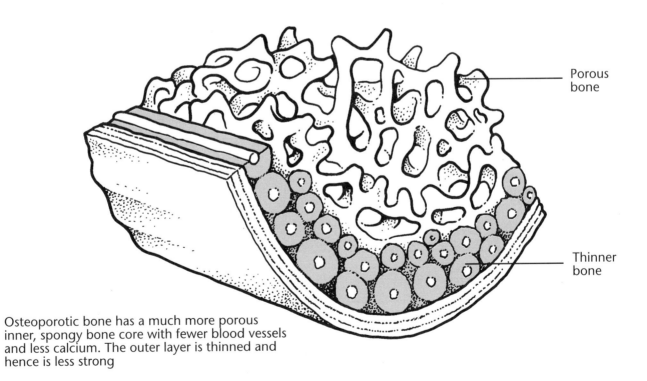

Porous bone

Osteoporotic bone has a much more porous inner, spongy bone core with fewer blood vessels and less calcium. The outer layer is thinned and hence is less strong

Thinner bone

Figure 22.3   Osteoporotic bone.

Osteoporosis references

This guideline is based on:
Breaking the Silence Initiative Guidelines on the Management of Osteoporosis (1994) developed by 24 physicians and written and produced by MEDIQ, 310 Regent St, London.

Compston JF (1992) Risk factors for osteoporosis. *Clin Endocrinol*: **36**; 223–4.

Consensus Development Conference (1993) Diagnosis, prophylaxis and treatment of osteoporosis. *Am J Med*: **94**; 646–50.

Cummings SR, Black DM, Nevitt MC *et al.* (1993) Bone density at various sites for prediction of hip fractures. *Lancet*: **341**; 72–5.

Diamond T, McGuigan L, Barbagallo S *et al.* (1995) Cyclical etidronate plus ergocalciferol prevents glucocorticoid induced bone loss in post-menopausal women. *Am J Med*: **98**; 459–63.

Grady D, Rubin S, Petitti DB *et al.* (1992) Hormone therapy to prevent disease and prolong life in postmenopausal women. *Ann Intern Med*: **117**; 1016–37.

Law M, Wald TJ and Meade TW (1991) Strategies for the prevention of osteoporosis and hip fracture. *BMJ*: **303**; 453–9.

Melton LJ, Eddy DM and Johnston CC (1990) Screening for osteoporosis. *Ann Intern Med*: **112**; 516–28.

Nordin REC (1994) Guidelines for bone densitometry. *Med J Aust*: **160**; 517–20.

Papapoulos SE, Landman JO, Bijvoet OLM *et al.* (1992) The use of bisphosphonates in the treatment of osteoporosis. *Bone*: **13**(Suppl. 1); S41–9.

Peel N and Eastell R (1995) ABC of rheumatology: osteoporosis. *BMJ*: **310**; 989–92.

Walsh LJ, Wong CA, Pringle M *et al.* (1996) Use of corticosteroids in the community and the prevention of secondary osteoporosis: a cross sectional study. *BMJ*: **313**; 344–6.

Watts NB, Harris ST, Genant HK *et al.* (1990) Intermittent cyclical etidronate treatment of postmenopausal osteoporosis. *N Engl J Med*: **323**; 73–9.

23

Otitis Media

Otitis media

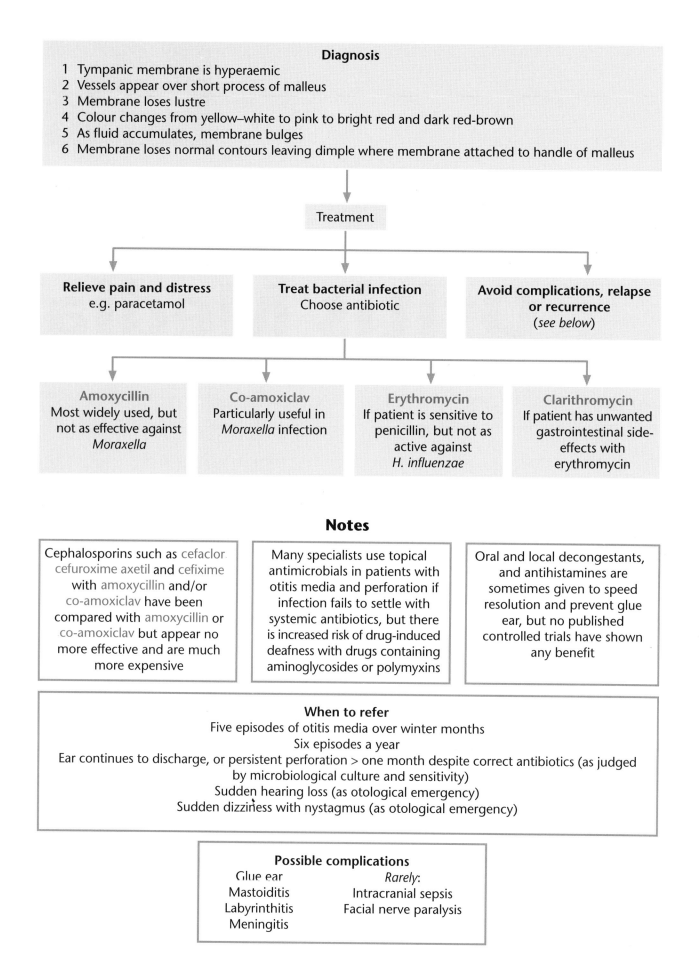

Diagnosis
1 Tympanic membrane is hyperaemic
2 Vessels appear over short process of malleus
3 Membrane loses lustre
4 Colour changes from yellow–white to pink to bright red and dark red-brown
5 As fluid accumulates, membrane bulges
6 Membrane loses normal contours leaving dimple where membrane attached to handle of malleus

Treatment

Relieve pain and distress
e.g. paracetamol

Treat bacterial infection
Choose antibiotic

Avoid complications, relapse or recurrence
(see below)

Amoxycillin
Most widely used, but not as effective against *Moraxella*

Co-amoxiclav
Particularly useful in *Moraxella* infection

Erythromycin
If patient is sensitive to penicillin, but not as active against *H. influenzae*

Clarithromycin
If patient has unwanted gastrointestinal side-effects with erythromycin

Notes

Cephalosporins such as cefaclor, cefuroxime axetil and cefixime with amoxycillin and/or co-amoxiclav have been compared with amoxycillin or co-amoxiclav but appear no more effective and are much more expensive

Many specialists use topical antimicrobials in patients with otitis media and perforation if infection fails to settle with systemic antibiotics, but there is increased risk of drug-induced deafness with drugs containing aminoglycosides or polymyxins

Oral and local decongestants, and antihistamines are sometimes given to speed resolution and prevent glue ear, but no published controlled trials have shown any benefit

When to refer
Five episodes of otitis media over winter months
Six episodes a year
Ear continues to discharge, or persistent perforation > one month despite correct antibiotics (as judged by microbiological culture and sensitivity)
Sudden hearing loss (as otological emergency)
Sudden dizziness with nystagmus (as otological emergency)

Possible complications
Glue ear	*Rarely*:
Mastoiditis	Intracranial sepsis
Labyrinthitis	Facial nerve paralysis
Meningitis	

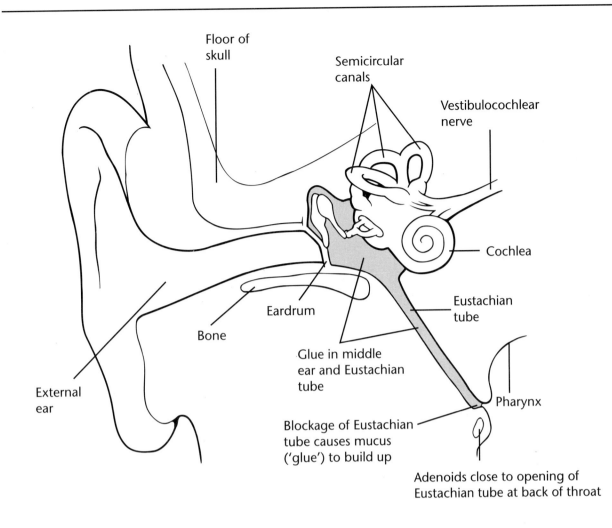

Figure 23.1   Glue ear.

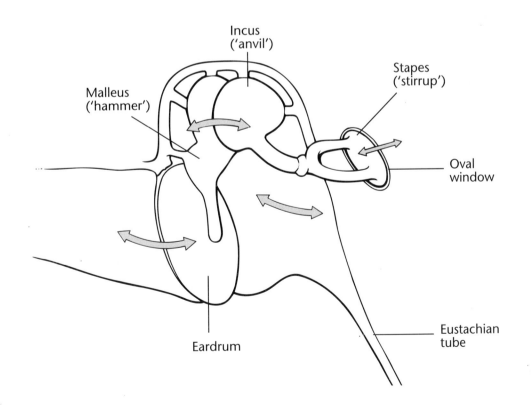

Figure 23.2   Movements of ossicles.

Otitis media references

This guideline is adapted from:
Management of acute otitis media and glue ear (1995) *Drug Therap Bull*: **33**; No. 2.

Bain J (1990) Justification for antibiotic use in general practice. *BMJ*: **300**; 1006–7.

Black NA, Sanderson CFB, Freeland AP *et al.* (1990) A randomised controlled trial of surgery for glue ear. *BMJ*: **300**; 1551–6.

Burke P, Bain J, Robinson D *et al.* (1991) Acute red ear in children: controlled trial of non-antibiotic treatment in general practice. *BMJ*: **303**; 558–62.

De Melker RA (1993) Treating persistent glue ear in children. *BMJ*: **306**; 5–6.

Dempster JH, Browning CG and Gatehouse SG (1993) A randomised study of the surgical management of children with persistent otitis media with effusion associated with hearing impairment. *J Laryngol Otol*: **107**; 284–9.

Ey JL, Holberg CJ, Aldous MB *et al.* (1995) Passive smoke exposure and otitis media in the first year of life. Group Health Medical Associates. *Pediatrics*: **95** (5); 670–7.

Hinton AE and Buckley G (1988) Parental smoking and middle ear effusions in children. *J Laryngol Otol*: **102**; 992–6.

Kaprio E, Haapaniemi J and Bondesson G (1988) Clinical efficacy of amoxycillin/clavulanic acid and cefaclor in acute otitis media. *Acta Otolaryngol (Stockh)*: **449**; 45–6.

Maw R and Bawden R (1993) Spontaneous resolution of severe chronic glue ear in children and the effect of adenoidectomy, tonsillectomy, and insertion of ventilation tubes (grommets). *BMJ*: **306**; 756–60.

Outcomes Department (1992) The treatment of glue ear in children. *Eff Health Care*: **4**; 1–16.

Williams RL, Chalmers TC, Stange KC *et al.* (1993) Use of antibiotics in preventing recurrent acute otitis media and in treating otitis media with effusion. *JAMA*: **270**; 1344–51.

24

Prostatic Hypertrophy

Benign prostatic hypertrophy

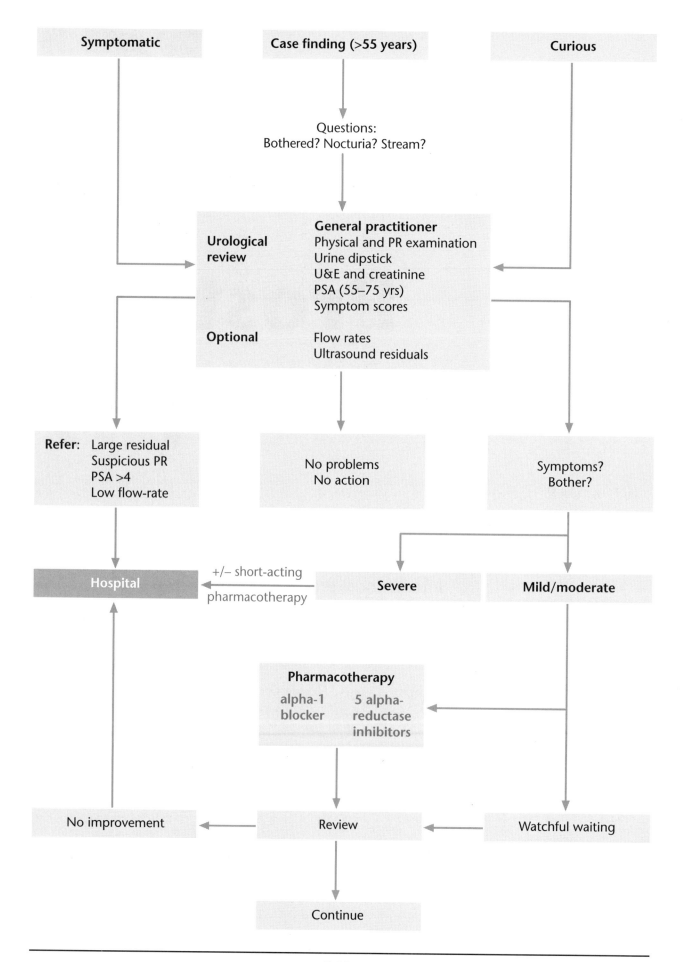

International prostate symptom scores (I-PSS)

		Not at all	Less than one time in five	Less than half the time	About half the time	More than half the time	Almost always
1	Over the past month, how often have you had a sensation of not emptying your bladder completely after you finished urinating?	0	1	2	3	4	5
2	Over the past month, how often have you had to urinate again less than two hours after you first urinated?	0	1	2	3	4	5
3	Over the past month, how often have you found you stopped and started again several times when you urinated?	0	1	2	3	4	5
4	Over the past month, how often have you found it difficult to postpone urination?	0	1	2	3	4	5
5	Over the past month, how often have you had a weak urinary stream?	0	1	2	3	4	5
6	Over the past month, how many times have you had to push or strain to begin urination?	0	1	2	3	4	5
		None	Once	Twice	Three times	Four times	>Five times
7	Over the past month, how many times did you most typically urinate from the time you went to bed at night to the time you got up in the morning?	0	1	2	3	4	5

Quality of life due to urinary symptoms

If you were to spend the rest of your life with your urinary condition just the way it is now, how would you feel about that? (This single question is recommended to assess the patient's own view of his quality of life. The question can be used to initiate a discussion.)	Delighted	0
	Pleased	1
	Mostly satisfied	2
	Mixed (about equally satisfied and dissatisfied)	3
	Mostly dissatisfied	4
	Unhappy	5
	Terrible	6

The international prostate symptom score (I-PSS)

The I-PSS has been developed to help evaluate the severity of symptoms caused by BPH. For each of the seven questions above, the patient may choose from six answers. Each answer is assigned points on a scale of 0 to 5. The total can therefore range from 0 to 35. As a guide, therefore:

Severity of symptoms

Mild   = 0 to 7
Moderate   = 8 to 19
Severe   = 20 to 35

It is recommended that the I-PSS and quality of life question be used at the initial consultation and after treatment to monitor process

Recording results

The I-PSS score and quality of life assessment index, L, should be noted periodically in the patient's medical records.

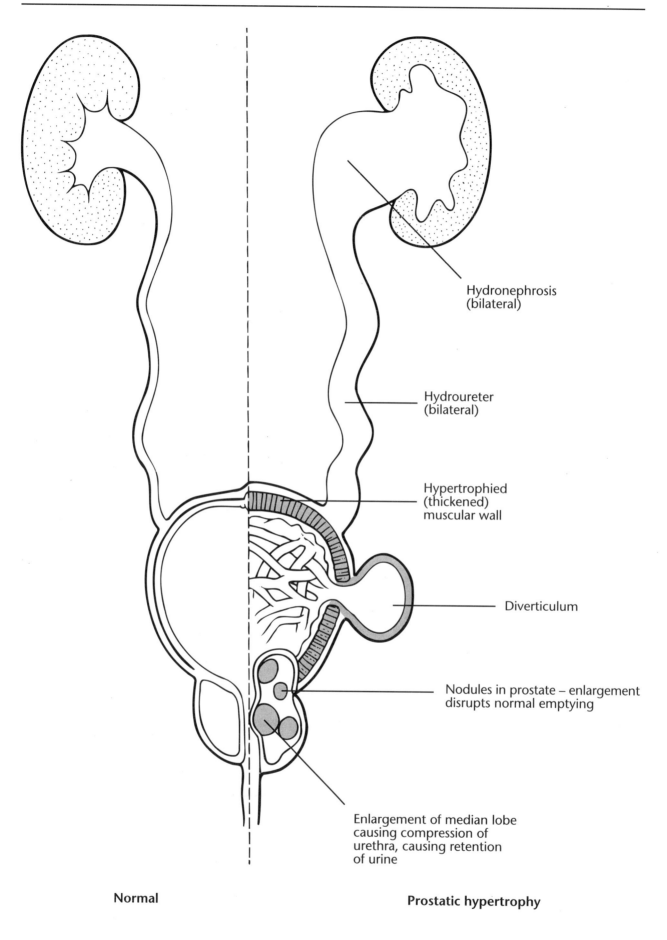

Hydronephrosis
(bilateral)

Hydroureter
(bilateral)

Hypertrophied
(thickened)
muscular wall

Diverticulum

Nodules in prostate – enlargement
disrupts normal emptying

Enlargement of median lobe
causing compression of
urethra, causing retention
of urine

Normal   **Prostatic hypertrophy**

Figure 24.1   Complications of benign prostatic hypertrophy.

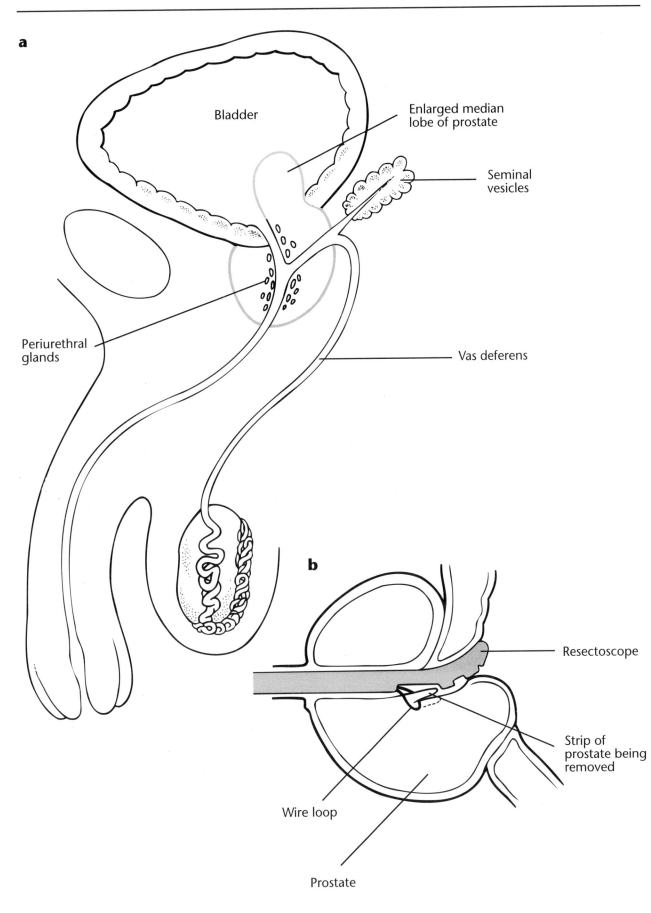

Figure 24.2 a Male genitalia with enlarged prostate gland; **b** Removal of hypertrophied prostate with resectoscope.

Benign prostatic hypertrophy references

This guideline is based on:
The WHO Consensus Guideline referred to in Cockett *et al.* (1991) below.

Bruskewitz RC (1992) Benign prostatic hyperplasia: drug and nondrug therapies. *Geriat*: **47**(12); 39–42.

Chapple C (1992) Medical treatment for benign prostatic hyperplasia [editorial]. *BMJ*: **304**; 1198–9.

Cockett AT, Aso Y, Denis L *et al.* (1991) World Health Organization Consensus Committee recommendations concerning the diagnosis of BPH. *Progres en Urologie*: **1**(6); 957–72.

Eri LM and Tveter KJ (1995) Alpha-blockade in the treatment of symptomatic benign prostatic hyperplasia. *J Urol*: **154**(3); 923–34.

Kirby RS (1994) Are the days of transurethral resection of prostate for benign prostatic hyperplasia numbered? Urologists must grasp the future. *BMJ*: **309**; 716–17.

Kreder KJ (1995) Combination drug therapy for benign prostatic hyperplasia. *JAMA*: **274**(4); 359.

Lepor H (1993) Medical therapy for benign prostatic hyperplasia. *Urol*: **42**(5); 483–501.

Lepor H (1996) The efficacy of terazosin and finasteride or both in benign prostatic hyperplasia. *N Engl J Med*: **335**; 533–9.

Lloyd SN, McMahon A, Muller W *et al.* (1994) Comparative study of selective alpha 1-adrenoceptor blockade versus surgery in the treatment of prostatic obstruction. *Brit J Urol*: **73**(6); 723.

McConnell JD (1995) Benign prostatic hyperplasia: treatment guidelines and patient classification. *Brit J Urol*: **76** (Suppl. 1); 129–46.

Nacey JN, Meffan PJ and Delahunt B (1995) The effect of finasteride on prostate volume, urinary flow rate and symptom score in men with benign prostatic hyperplasia. *Austral NZ J Surg*: **65**(1); 35–9.

Oesterling JE (1995) Benign prostatic hyperplasia. Medical and minimally invasive treatment options. *New Engl J Med*: **332**(2); 99–109.

Rhinitis

Treatment of allergic rhinitis

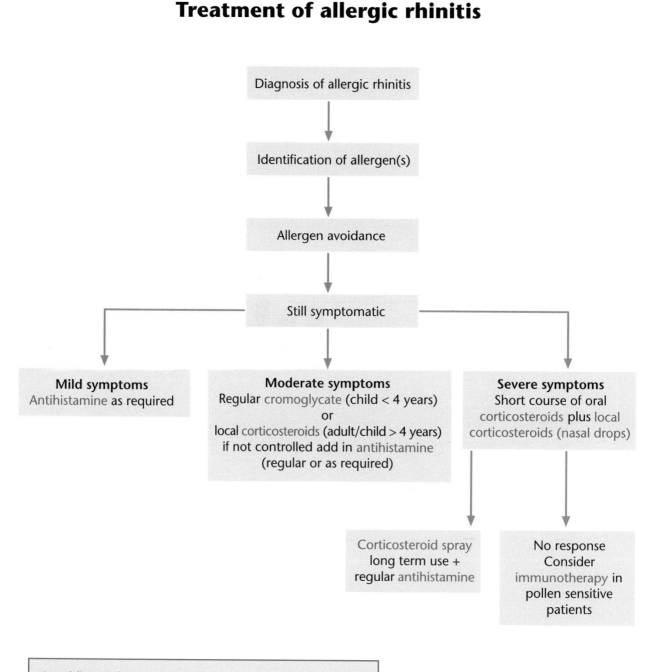

Diagnosis of allergic rhinitis

↓

Identification of allergen(s)

↓

Allergen avoidance

↓

Still symptomatic

Mild symptoms
Antihistamine as required

Moderate symptoms
Regular cromoglycate (child < 4 years)
or
local corticosteroids (adult/child > 4 years)
if not controlled add in antihistamine
(regular or as required)

Severe symptoms
Short course of oral
corticosteroids plus local
corticosteroids (nasal drops)

Corticosteroid spray
long term use +
regular antihistamine

No response
Consider
immunotherapy in
pollen sensitive
patients

In addition: short courses of intranasal decongestants
may be needed
(i) at the start of treatment
(ii) for flying
(iii) in the 'thick phase' of upper respiratory tract infections

Treatment failure
Review diagnosis
Review compliance
Query infection or structural problems

Watery rhinorrhoea
Try anticholingeric
Ipratropium spray

Matching medication to symptoms

	Sneezing	Discharge	Blockage	Anosmia
Cromoglycate	++	+	+	−
Decongestant	−	−	+++	−
Antihistamine	+++	++	+/−	−
Ipratropium	−	++	−	−
Topical steroids	+++	++	++	+
Oral steroids	++	++	+++	++

After Mygind N (1992) *Rhinology*. Surgical supplement.

Rhinitis references

This guideline is based on:
Scadding G, Drake-Lee A, Durham S *et al.* (1995) *Rhinitis Management Guidelines.*
British Society for Allergy and Clinical Immunology.

Acquadro MA and Montgomery WW (1996) Treatment of chronic paranasal sinus pain and minimal sinus disease. *Ann Otol Rhinol Laryngol*: **105**(8); 607–14.

Anonymous (1995) Fluticasone propionate nasal spray for allergic rhinitis [medical letter]. *Drugs & Therapeutics*: **37**(940); 5–6.

Bronsky EA, Dockhorn RJ, Meltzer EO *et al.* (1996) Fluticasone propionate aqueous nasal spray compared with terfenadine tablets in the treatment of seasonal allergic rhinitis. *J Allergy Clin Immunol*: **97**(4); 915–21.

Graft DF (1996) Allergic and nonallergic rhinitis. Directing medical therapy at specific symptoms [review]. *Postgrad Med*: **100**(2); 64–9, 73–4.

Grossman J, Banov C, Boggs P (1995) *et al.* Use of ipratropium bromide nasal spray in chronic treatment of nonallergic perennial rhinitis, alone and in combination with other perennial rhinitis medications. *J Allergy Clin Immunol*: **95** (5 Pt 2); 1123–7.

Guarderas JC (1996) Rhinitis and sinusitis: office management [review]. *Mayo Clinic Proceed*: **71**(9); 882–8.

Harvey RP, Comer C, Sanders B *et al.* (1996) Model for outcomes assessment of antihistamine use for seasonal allergic rhinitis. *J Allergy Clin Immunol*: **97**(6); 1233–41.

International Rhinitis Management Working Group (1994) International consensus report on the diagnosis and management of rhinitis. *J Allergy Clin Immunol*: **19** (Suppl.).

Jorres R, Nowak D and Magnussen H (1996) The effect of ozone exposure on allergen responsiveness in subjects with asthma or rhinitis. *Am J Respir Crit Care Med*: **153**(1); 56–64.

Li CS and Hsu LY (1996) Home dampness and childhood respiratory symptoms in a subtropical climate. *Arch Environ Health*: **51**(1); 42–6.

Meltzer EO, Weiler JM and Widlitz MD (1996) Comparative outdoor study of the efficacy, onset and duration of action, and safety of cetirizine, loratadine, and placebo for seasonal allergic rhinitis. *J Allergy Clin Immunol*: **97**(2); 617–26.

Prenner BM, Chervinsky P, Hampel FC Jr *et al.* (1996) Double-strength beclomethasone dipropionate (84 micrograms spray) aqueous nasal spray in the treatment of seasonal allergic rhinitis. *J Allergy Clin Immunol*: **98**(2); 302–8.

26

Urinary Tract Infection

Urinary tract infection

Simple UTI in non-elderly females

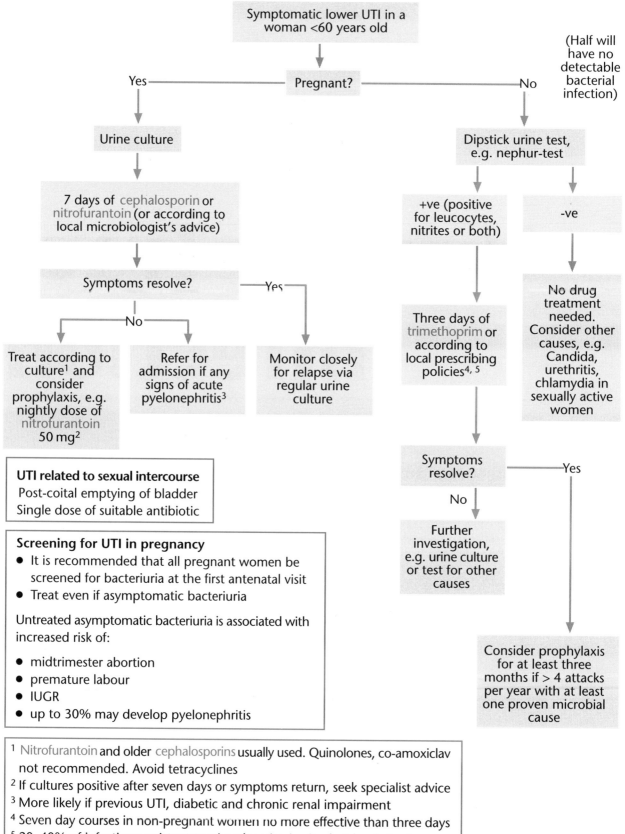

Symptomatic lower UTI in a woman <60 years old

Pregnant?

Yes ———————— No

(Half will have no detectable bacterial infection)

Yes branch:

Urine culture

7 days of cephalosporin or nitrofurantoin (or according to local microbiologist's advice)

Symptoms resolve? ———— Yes

No:

Treat according to culture[1] and consider prophylaxis, e.g. nightly dose of nitrofurantoin 50 mg[2]

Refer for admission if any signs of acute pyelonephritis[3]

Yes:

Monitor closely for relapse via regular urine culture

No branch:

Dipstick urine test, e.g. nephur-test

+ve (positive for leucocytes, nitrites or both)

-ve

Three days of trimethoprim or according to local prescribing policies[4, 5]

No drug treatment needed. Consider other causes, e.g. Candida, urethritis, chlamydia in sexually active women

Symptoms resolve? ———— Yes

No

Further investigation, e.g. urine culture or test for other causes

Consider prophylaxis for at least three months if > 4 attacks per year with at least one proven microbial cause

---

UTI related to sexual intercourse
Post-coital emptying of bladder
Single dose of suitable antibiotic

Screening for UTI in pregnancy
- It is recommended that all pregnant women be screened for bacteriuria at the first antenatal visit
- Treat even if asymptomatic bacteriuria

Untreated asymptomatic bacteriuria is associated with increased risk of:

- midtrimester abortion
- premature labour
- IUGR
- up to 30% may develop pyelonephritis

---

[1] Nitrofurantoin and older cephalosporins usually used. Quinolones, co-amoxiclav not recommended. Avoid tetracyclines

[2] If cultures positive after seven days or symptoms return, seek specialist advice

[3] More likely if previous UTI, diabetic and chronic renal impairment

[4] Seven day courses in non-pregnant women no more effective than three days

[5] 20–40% of infections resistant to trimethoprim *in vitro* but levels *in vivo* are higher, so most will respond

Complicated urinary tract infections

Complicated UTI if it affects the following groups

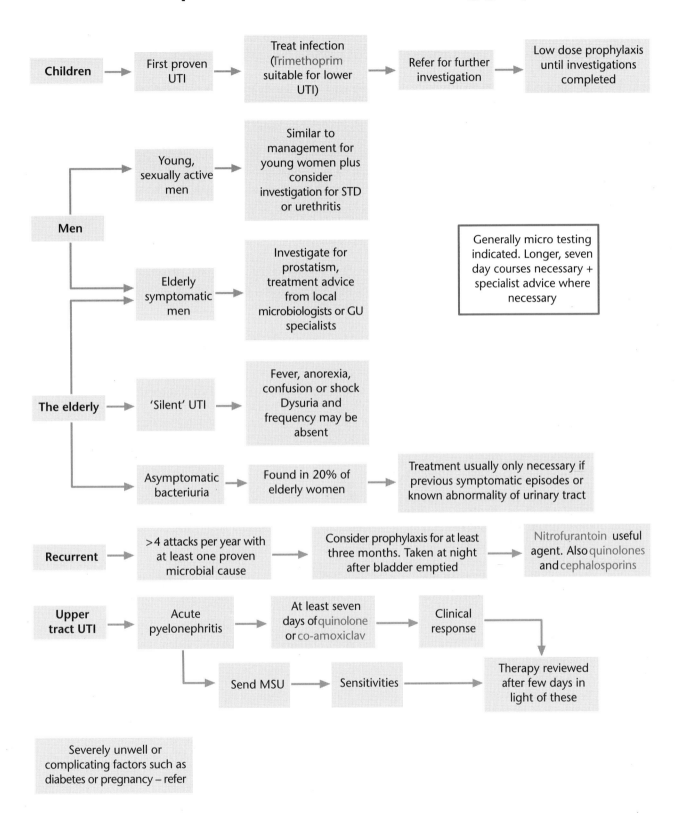

Children → First proven UTI → Treat infection (Trimethoprim suitable for lower UTI) → Refer for further investigation → Low dose prophylaxis until investigations completed

Men
→ Young, sexually active men → Similar to management for young women plus consider investigation for STD or urethritis
→ Elderly symptomatic men → Investigate for prostatism, treatment advice from local microbiologists or GU specialists

Generally micro testing indicated. Longer, seven day courses necessary + specialist advice where necessary

The elderly
→ 'Silent' UTI → Fever, anorexia, confusion or shock Dysuria and frequency may be absent
→ Asymptomatic bacteriuria → Found in 20% of elderly women → Treatment usually only necessary if previous symptomatic episodes or known abnormality of urinary tract

Recurrent → >4 attacks per year with at least one proven microbial cause → Consider prophylaxis for at least three months. Taken at night after bladder emptied → Nitrofurantoin useful agent. Also quinolones and cephalosporins

Upper tract UTI → Acute pyelonephritis → At least seven days of quinolone or co-amoxiclav → Clinical response → Therapy reviewed after few days in light of these
→ Send MSU → Sensitivities → Therapy reviewed after few days in light of these

Severely unwell or complicating factors such as diabetes or pregnancy – refer

Urinary tract infection references

This guideline is based on:
Medicine Resources Centre (1995) UTI guidelines. *MeReC Bulletin.* 6(8).

Anon (1995) Thorough investigation and treatment reduces risks of bacteriuria in pregnancy. *Drugs Ther Perspect*: **1**; 10–11.

Anon (1995) Revised indications for co-trimoxazole. *Current Problems*: **21**; 6.

Bint AJ and Hill D (1994) Bacteriuria of pregnancy – an update on significance, diagnosis and management. *J Antimicrob Chemother*: **33** (Suppl. A); 93–7.

Briggs GG, Freeman RK and Yaffe SJ (1994) *Drugs in pregnancy and lactation* (Fourth edn). Williams & Wilkins, pp 808–13.

Brumfitt W and Hamilton-Miller JMT (1994) Consensus viewpoint on management of urinary infections. *J Antimicrob Chemother*: **33** (Suppl. A); 147–53.

Dearden A and Williams JD (1995) Urinary tract infection in adults. *Medicine*: **23**; 177–83.

Hatton J, Hughes M and Raymond CH (1994) Management of bacterial urinary tract infections in adults. *Ann Pharmacother*: **28**; 1264–72.

Merrick MV, Notghi A, Chalmers N *et al.* (1995) Long-term follow up to determine the prognostic value of imaging after urinary tract infections. Part 1: Reflux. *Arch Dis Child*: **72**(5); 388–92.

Merrick MV, Notghi A, Chalmers N *et al.* (1995) Long-term follow up to determine the prognostic value of imaging after urinary tract infections. Part 2: Scarring. *Arch Dis Child*: **72**(5); 393–6.

Report of physicians at the Hospital for Sick Children, Great Ormond Street, London [clinical conference] (1996) Vesicoureteric reflux: all in the genes? *Lancet*: **348**; 725–8.

Welsby P (1995) Treatment and prevention of urinary tract infections. *Prescriber*: 5 July; 25–42.

Wilkie ME, Almond MK and Marsh FP (1992) Diagnosis and management of urinary tract infections in adults. *BMJ*: **305**; 1137–41.